D1550080

Healthcare Interpreting

Benjamins Current Topics

Special issues of established journals tend to circulate within the orbit of the subscribers of those journals. For the Benjamins Current Topics series a number of special issues have been selected containing salient topics of research with the aim to widen the readership and to give this interesting material an additional lease of life in book format.

Volume 9

Healthcare Interpreting. Discourse and Interaction
Edited by Franz Pöchhacker and Miriam Shlesinger

These materials were previously published in *Interpreting* 7:2 (2005)

Healthcare Interpreting

Discourse and Interaction

Edited by

Franz Pöchhacker
University of Vienna

Miriam Shlesinger
Bar-Ilan University

John Benjamins Publishing Company
Amsterdam / Philadelphia

The paper used in this publication meets the minimum requirements of
American National Standard for Information Sciences – Permanence of
Paper for Printed Library Materials, ANSI z39.48-1984.

Library of Congress Cataloging-in-Publication Data

Healthcare interpreting : discourse and interaction / edited by Franz Pöchhacker, Miriam
    Shlesinger.
    p. ; cm. -- (Benjamins current topics, ISSN 1874-0081 ; v. 9)
Includes bibliographical references.
1. Medicine--Translating. 2. Health facilities--Translating services. 3. Physician and
    patient. I. Pöchhacker, Franz. II. Shlesinger, Miriam, 1947- III. Series.
[DNLM: 1. Professional-Patient Relations. 2. Translating. 3. Communication Barriers.
    W 62 H4347 2007]
R119.5.H43   2007
362.1--dc22   2007007385
ISBN 978-90-272-2239-8 (alk. paper)

John Benjamins Publishing Co. · P.O. Box 36224 · 1020 ME Amsterdam · The Netherlands
John Benjamins North America · P.O. Box 27519 · Philadelphia PA 19118-0519 · USA

Table of contents

About the Authors

Yvan Leanza has a degree in psychology, including clinical training, and holds a PhD in educational sciences from the University of Geneva. He has done research on the acculturation processes of migrants and on healthcare professionals working with "different" clients. His PhD research focused on Swiss pediatricians working with families from Kosovo and Sri Lanka. As a postdoctoral fellow (on a grant from the Swiss National Science Foundation) in the Division of Social and Transcultural Psychiatry and at the Department of Family Medicine at McGill University, Montreal, he continues his work on interpreting and on the relation to the Other in medical settings.

Authors' address: Faculté de psychologie et des sciences de l'éducation · Université de Genève
42, bvd du Pont d'Arve · CH–1211 Genève 4 · Suisse
E-mail: Yvan.Leanza@pse.unige.ch

Carmen Valero Garcés, PhD, is Associate Professor of English at the University of Alcalá de Henares (Madrid), Spain, where she coordinates the FITISPos research group on community interpreting and translation (CI&T) and directs the postgraduate and undergraduate programs in CI&T. She has organized two international conferences on community interpreting and translation at Alcalá (2002, 2005) and edited the proceedings. She has also published several books and many articles related to cross-cultural communication, interpreting and translating, second language acquisition and contrastive linguistics.
Website: http://www2.uah.es/traduccion

Author's address: Department of Modern Languages · University of Alcalá · C/ Trinidad 5 · 28801 Alcalá de Henares (Madrid) · Spain
E-mail: mcarmen.valero@uah.es

Friedel Dubslaff is Associate Professor of interpreting at the Aarhus School of Business, Denmark. She graduated in languages from the University of Hamburg, Germany (1970), and holds an MA in German from the University of Aarhus, Denmark (1979). In 1996 she received her PhD with a dissertation on simultaneous interpreting at the Aarhus School of Business. Academic interests: interpreting research (conference and community interpreting), translation, text linguistics.

Further field of interest: professionalization of community interpreting in migrant languages in Denmark.

Bodil Martinsen is an Associate Professor at the Aarhus School of Business, Denmark. She holds an MA (LSP) in French (Interpreting and Translation) from the Aarhus School of Business. She is a State-authorized Interpreter and Translator and works as a freelance court interpreter and translator. Academic interests: interpreting research (community interpreting with special reference to legal interpreting). Further field of interest: professionalization of community interpreting in migrant languages in Denmark.

Authors' addresses: Department of Language and Business Communication · Aarhus School of Business ·Fuglesangs Allé 4 · DK–8210 Aarhus V · Denmark
E-mail: fd@asb.dk, brm@asb.dk

Hanneke Bot holds a Masters degree in rural sociology and is a Dutch government registered psychotherapist. She works in a clinic for the psychiatric treatment of asylum seekers and refugees in the Netherlands. She works with interpreters on a daily basis. Her PhD research on working with interpreters in mental health was published by Rodopi in 2005.

Author's address: De Gelderse Roos / Phoenix · P.O. Box 27 · 6870 AA Renkum · The Netherlands
E-mail: h.bot@degelderseroos.nl

Raffaela Merlini is Associate Professor of English Language and Translation at the University of Macerata, Italy. She teaches simultaneous and consecutive interpreting from English into Italian at the School of Modern Languages for Interpreters and Translators (SSLMIT) of the University of Trieste, Italy. She was Head of the Italian Section in the Department of Modern Languages at the University of Salford, England, where she lectured from 1996 to 1999. Merlini has published in the field of interpreting studies, particularly on consecutive and dialogue interpreting topics. She has worked as a conference interpreter in high-level institutional settings.

Roberta Favaron is employed as full-time Italian-English hospital interpreter at ISMETT (*Mediterranean Institute for Transplantation and Specialized Therapies*) in Palermo, Italy. She graduated from the School of Modern Languages for Interpreters and Translators (SSLMIT) of the University of Trieste, Italy, where she worked as lecturer in Italian to foreign students and researcher in the field of dubbing and subtitling from September 2002 to August 2004. She has published in the field of medical interpreting.

Authors' address: SSLMIT, University of Trieste · Via Fabio Filzi, 14 · 34135 Trieste ·Italy
E-mail: rmerlini@units.it · rfavaron@ismett.edu

Introduction

Discourse-based research on healthcare interpreting

One of the most remarkable developments in interpreting studies since the mid-1990s has been the emergence of community interpreting as an increasingly significant field of professional practice and academic research. Among the various institutional settings in which community interpreters work, the field of health care is of particular importance. Aside from legal settings and educational interpreting for the Deaf, medical settings probably constitute the most prevalent field of practice for interpreters in the community. It was in the field of health care that some of the earliest initiatives for the provision of community interpreting services were taken (e.g. the Hospital Interpreter Service established in New South Wales, Australia, in 1974), and it was medical interpreters who, in the 1990s, formed the first professional organizations for community-based interpreting outside the judicial domain. As mediated communication in healthcare settings slowly gained visibility, it also came to attract the attention of scholars interested in interpreting. Among the first to focus on interpreter-mediated medical encounters was Cecilia Wadensjö (1992), whose corpus of Russian-Swedish dialogue interpreting included 13 interactions involving nurses or doctors in healthcare or childcare clinics. Her discourse-based research approach, presented most authoritatively in Wadensjö (1998), proved highly influential to the field of interpreting studies in general, informing a distinct paradigm centered on **dialogic discourse** in **triadic interaction** (see Pöchhacker 2004: 79).

Wadensjö's influence on dialogue interpreting research is particularly evident in the papers brought together in this volume. What is less evident is her role in the genesis of these contributions, all of which were presented at the Fourth Critical Link Conference in Stockholm in May 2004, organized by a team including Birgitta Englund Dimitrova and Cecilia Wadensjö. Three of the papers presented here even come from the same conference session, "Empirical Research on Healthcare Encounters", which took place on May 23, 2004. Moreover, these papers are strikingly close in thematic and methodological orientation, drawing on discourse-analytical frameworks to analyze mediated interaction in healthcare settings. Indeed, it is this – coincidental – relatedness that gave rise to the idea of publishing these papers as a special issue of the journal *Interpreting* (vol. 7, no. 2, 2005), now made available in the Benjamins Current Topics series.

The five papers from the Critical Link Conference thus have two interrelated focal points, as reflected in the title of this book: one is the discourse-based analysis of interpreter-mediated interaction, and the other, on a broader level, is (cross-cultural) communication in healthcare settings. In this sense, the present volume is one of the first collections of researchdevoted to interpreting in health care. While we consider it highly appropriate and timely to accord this topic special attention, we also realize that the present set of papers covers only a fraction of what a publication on healthcare interpreting research might address. (For a more extensive review with a focus on methodological issues, see Pöchhacker 2006.) Before introducing the collection as such, we would therefore like to contextualize this set of papers within the much more comprehensive and varied literature on medical interpreting, highlighting their specificity as well as their contribution and relationship to the broader picture.

Researchers in interpreting studies have not been among the first to recognize the significance of medical interpreting as a field of practice and research. Rather, it was in the health and social sciences and, occasionally, in linguistic disciplines that studies on interpreters in health care were carried out several decades before the topic was given international attention at the First Critical Link Conference in 1995. In one of the earliest contributions, published in *Mental Hygiene*, Bloom et al. (1966) sketched out three different interpreter roles in interviewing. On the basis of illustrative vignettes of authentic interview situations, they suggested that the interpreter may either take over the interview, serve as a mere tool to facilitate communication or work in partnership with the interviewing specialist. All of these three options have proven significant in the debate on interpreter use in health care, and the issue of the interpreter's role has been paramount throughout (see, for instance, Drennan & Swartz 1999).

A specialty within health care in which interpreting has been given particular attention is mental health. One of the earliest studies was reported by Price (1975), who conducted a quantitative analysis of psychiatric interviews with Hindustani-speaking patients in which three different interpreters (two orderlies and a patient in remission) worked with each of three English-speaking doctors. Assessing both translational accuracy and the interpreters' linguistic proficiency, Price found a higher rate of various mistranslations (omissions, distorted questions, additions, etc.) in the performances of the two orderlies (with considerable experience in interpreting) than in the renditions by the better-educated patient serving as interpreter. Aside from a high rate of omissions in relaying patients' answers to the psychiatrist, the author also found clinically significant additions, e.g. in a patient's description of hallucinatory voices, and concluded that "an interpreter's apparent competence may readily be mistaken for true competence" (1975: 263).

In an analysis conducted from a linguistic rather than a medical background, Lang (1975) investigated the performance of orderlies serving as interpreters for Enga and Tok Pisin in Papua New Guinea. Adopting a qualitative, discourse-based approach, Lang illustrated various types of mistranslation (additions and omissions) and discussed the interpreters' behavior with reference to professional interpreting standards ("taught in interpreter training schools in Europe"). As in the study by Price (1975), Lang (1975) found an asymmetrical pattern of deviations in the rendition of doctors' vs. patients' utterances, and many instances of the orderly assuming an active third-party role.

Similar findings were published in the *British Medical Journal* by Launer (1978), who analyzed tape-recorded consultations between 30 Hausa-speaking patients and four English-speaking doctors mediated by seven medical orderlies in a Nigerian hospital. He noted numerous deviations from the standard of accurate and complete ("word-for-word") translation, and found that "interpreters were inclined to conduct much of the consultations themselves" (Launer 1978: 934).

These few early studies on interpreters in health care, by medical specialists and linguists, serve to indicate some of the main themes and lines of investigation in this field. In essence, all of these studies are founded upon a record of the interacting parties' utterances, of their "discourse", in the more specific sense of "language use in social interaction" (van Dijk 1997). Using audio-recordings and more or less complete transcriptions thereof, researchers have analyzed such discourse data both quantitatively and qualitatively, foregrounding a number of different research issues. Among the earliest concerns is the accuracy and completeness of the interpreters' renditions, and the nature of any "deviations" or errors. Apart from the studies mentioned earlier, a much-cited example from the medical literature is the report by Ebden et al. (1988) in *The Lancet* on translation errors in bilingual consultations in which relatives accompanying Gujarati-speaking patients served as interpreters in an English hospital. A more recent and comprehensive study was reported by Flores et al. (2003), who analyzed thirteen pediatric encounters in which communication with Spanish-speaking patients was mediated by (largely untrained) hospital interpreters as well as ad hoc interpreters (nurse, social worker, sibling). The authors found numerous instances of omission, substitution and editorialization, two thirds of which were judged to be of potential clinical significance and were found significantly more often in the performance of ad hoc interpreters.

Alongside this first major line of investigation, which focuses on errors in the interpreting product and on their clinical significance, has been the concern with the interactional role of persons serving as interpreters, as raised in some of the earliest papers cited above. The issue of role descriptions and expectations, a quintessential topic of sociology, has been addressed not so much by medical researchers and linguists as by researchers with a background in interpreting or in the social sciences. Groundbreaking work in this regard was done by medical anthropologists such as Joseph Kaufert and associates (e.g. Kaufert & Koolage 1984), who highlighted the cultural complexities involved in the interpreter's task. The crucial issue of the interpreter's role, as captured in notions such as "cultural brokering" or "visibility", emerged as a distinct thematic orientation in which research is mainly founded on sociological and sociolinguistic approaches. Two complementary dimensions can be identified in this line of work: survey research, based on questionnaires (e.g. Pöchhacker 2000a; Angelelli 2004) or interviews (e.g. Allaoui 2005), and discourse-based analyses of the micro-sociology of interaction (e.g. Wadensjö 1998, 2001; Metzger 1999). The latter corresponds to the approach taken by the authors in this volume.

Another fundamental concern that has been addressed primarily with concepts and tools drawn from the social sciences is the institutional status of the interpreter in medical settings. "Who interprets?" is a basic research question that has been dealt with in a number of surveys to assess communicative practices and interpreting needs in healthcare institutions (e.g. Ginsberg et al. 1995; Pöchhacker 2000b; Bischoff & Loutan 2004). These quantitative studies have yielded findings from the point of view of healthcare service providers, whereas the clients' perspective, in community interpreting in general, has received rather less attention (but see Edwards et al. 2005).

Research on communicative practices and policies in various healthcare institutions has yielded an uneven picture. As pointed out two decades ago by Putsch (1985: 3344), "Institutions vary in their arrangements to meet the needs of monolingual patients and health care providers. Even when there is a well-described need, many facilities have not dealt with language and cultural problems in a formal operational sense." While this statement may still apply in a great many national and legal contexts, there have also been major initiatives for ensuring "culturally sensitive care", including specific arrangements such as over-the-phone interpreting, in-house interpreter pools and remote simultaneous interpretation, all of which merit, and indeed require, further investigation. From the perspective of the healthcare system, these communicative arrangements prompt some critical questions regarding their respective effect on medical service provision. Indeed, such issues as equitable access to services, liability in case of miscommunication, effective service delivery, cost efficiency, quality of care, and patient satisfaction have come to be addressed by a growing body of research in the medical sciences. Ever since the much-noted review article by Woloshin et al. (1995), which appeared in the *Journal of the American Medical Association* in the year of the First Critical Link Conference, studies on the problems and effects of language barriers in medicine have become increasingly numerous. Reviewing this growing body of research reports in medical journals would clearly be beyond the scope of this introduction; fortunately, some 135 of them have been made accessible in an annotated bibliography published in 2001. But as noted by the compilers (cf. Jacobs et al. 2003: 2), the notion of "interpreter use" in some of these medical studies is defined very broadly and does not necessarily distinguish between ad hoc interpreting by accompanying persons or bilingual staff, and "professional" interpreting, the latter usually referring to "paid" interpreters, but not necessarily to "trained" or particularly qualified ones.

This lack of attention to the implications of an interpreter's competence and performance standards reflects an insufficient degree of interdisciplinary exchange and cooperation between research in medicine and interpreting studies. This holds true both for work on the medical and institutional dimensions of healthcare service **provision** and for the (much less numerous) analyses of the interpreting **product**. While it is true that the topic of communication in medicine has gained enormous momentum since the late 1990s – as reflected in training initiatives and international conferences, the issue of language barriers and interpreter use seems to be a marginal concern, if it comes up in these contexts at all. Thirty years ago, Lang (1975: 172) observed that "in the field of doctor-patient interaction language problems are customarily ignored entirely". While progress has undoubtedly been made toward eliminating this blind spot, the medical literature as a whole, where it addresses problems of language and communication at all, is still far from treating foreign-language barriers as a mainstream concern.

The same can be said about medical communication studies as grounded in discourse analysis, pragmatics and sociolinguistics. Judging from the inaugural editorial of *Communication & Medicine*, a new "interdisciplinary journal of healthcare, ethics and society" (Sarangi 2004), the significance of language barriers and the implications of mediated communication have yet to be recognized fully by communication scholars and by medical researchers. And yet, discourse analysts and sociolinguists of various persuasions have clearly been highly influential in the study of interpreted healthcare encounters. The analysis of interpreting **performance** based on transcripts of authentic discourse represents an essential line of work, pursued by healthcare researchers and linguists as well as specialists in interpreting.

The papers in this volume are typical of this methodological orientation and highlight both the diversity of disciplinary approaches and the significant common ground shared by those studying discourse and interaction in healthcare settings. With regard to disciplinary perspectives, two of the contributions are by professionals with a clinical background (in psychology and psychotherapy), and three are by specialists in linguistics and interpreting. The five articles cover a number of settings and specialties, from general medicine to pediatrics, psychiatry and speech therapy, and the discourse-based analyses feature languages such as Arabic, Dari, Farsi, Italian and Spanish in combination with Danish, Dutch, English and French. Aside from Wadensjö's (1992, 1998) groundbreaking work and the Goffmanian notion of "footing", authors draw on sources from various theoretical frameworks and from such analytical approaches as conversation analysis and institutional discourse analysis.

This conspicuous variety even within a well-defined line of research makes it difficult (and then again, easy) to arrange the five papers in a coherent sequence. Each of them is substantial and multi-faceted enough to stand on its own and, at the same time, link up with the others in multiple ways. In the following brief introduction of the individual pieces (over and above the information found in the respective abstracts), our rationale for the arrangement we have chosen should also become clear.

The first paper, by Yvan **Leanza**, brings perhaps the most comprehensive perspective to the topic of mediated medical encounters, despite its focus on the domain of pediatrics. Contextualizing his work with reference to both the "biomedical literature" and the more theoretical social-science contributions ("voice of medicine" vs. "voice of the lifeworld"), Leanza triangulates observation, interview data and discourse transcripts, and presents both qualitative data and quantitative findings. Incorporating some lesser-known francophone publications on the subject, his exploration of the interpreter's role(s) in the interaction from several vantage points broadly sets the stage for the more strictly discourse-oriented papers to follow.

The wide-ranging account by Carmen **Valero** of characteristic features in dyadic versus triadic doctor-patient consultations illustrates how communicative limitations and interpreters' performance standards manifest themselves in the interactive discourse. Among other things, she shows how unmediated (monolingual) consultations involving limited-proficiency patients share some traits with encounters mediated by an ad hoc interpreter. Again, the corpus of authentic discourse data (two consultations each for three types of communicative constellation: no interpreter, ad hoc interpreter, trained interpreter) is subjected to some quantitative analysis to complement the illustrative excerpts.

A corpus that is particularly well-suited to quantification is examined by Friedel **Dubslaff** and Bodil **Martinsen** for interpreters' use of direct versus indirect speech, often cited as an indicator of professional versus lay or ad hoc interpreting. In four simulated doctor-patient interviews based on the same script, the untrained practitioners participating in an examination session are found to adopt different styles of address and to struggle even with non-specialized medical terms. These difficulties are often linked with certain pronoun shifts indicating changes of footing.

Different forms of address (direct vs. indirect style) and various types of footings are explored in greater detail in the two remaining papers, both of which focus on specific healthcare settings. In a more qualitative and theoretically framed account of pronoun use, psychotherapist Hanneke **Bot** analyzes six interpreter-mediated therapy sessions and identifies four types of changes in perspective, including the previously unexplored strategy of "direct representation" as a specific style of reported speech.

Last, but by no means least, Raffaela **Merlini** and Roberta **Favaron** present an in-depth analysis of three professionally interpreted speech pathology sessions. Based on their qualitative study of such discourse features as turn-taking, topic development, choice of footing, additions and prosody, the authors frame the complexity of interpreter behavior as the "voice of interpreting", fluctuating between the voices of medicine and of the lifeworld. Based on the three interactions under study, Merlini and Favaron conclude that going beyond the idealized professional style of formal and detached interpreting may serve to strengthen the "voice of the lifeworld", thus linking back up with the stance adopted in the first paper by Leanza.

As regards the form of the five papers brought together here, no attempt was made to impose a uniform style for transcription and presentation of examples from the corpus. In every case, though, the English interlinear translation appears in italics underneath the respective original utterance in standard font.

Rounding off the set of five articles in this journal-based volume are three book reviews. The first presents publications by Carmen Valero relating to the more comprehensive domain of community or public-service interpreting; the second, on the published doctoral dissertation by Bernd Meyer, introduces a discourse-analytical framework used by German scholars to study interpreting in medical communication; and the third reviews two volumes by Claudia Angelelli with a distinct focus on medical interpreting.

As mentioned at the outset of this Introduction, this publication would not have been possible without the active support of Birgitta Englund Dimitrova and Cecilia Wadensjö, both of whom are members of the editorial board of *Interpreting*. They would have deserved credit as guest editors of this collection, had it not been for their heavy workload as co-editors of the Critical Link conference proceedings, which this set of papers could be seen to complement.

We are also grateful to our contributors for agreeing to have their work published here, and for investing much time and effort in the course of the peer-review and revision process. These published versions of five Critical Link conference contributions cover some significant ground in a much wider and highly interdisciplinary field. It is our hope that this collection may stimulate further work to explore the field of healthcare interpreting more fully.

Franz Pöchhacker and Miriam Shlesinger

References

Allaoui, R. (2005). *Dolmetschen im Krankenhaus. Rollenerwartungen und Rollenverständnisse.* Göttingen: Cuvillier.

Angelelli, C. V. (2004). *Revisiting the interpreter's role.* Amsterdam/Philadelphia: John Benjamins.

Bischoff, A. & Loutan, L. (2004). Interpreting in Swiss hospitals. *Interpreting* 6 (2), 181–204.

Bloom, M., Hanson, H., Frires, G. & South, V. (1966). The use of interpreters in interviewing. *Mental Hygiene* 50, 214–221.

Drennan, G. & Swartz, L. (1999). A concept over-burdened: Institutional roles for psychiatric interpreters in post-apartheid South Africa. *Interpreting* 4 (2), 169–198.

Ebden, P., Bhatt, A., Carey, O. J. & Harrison, B. (1988). The bilingual consultation. *The Lancet*, February 13, 1988, 347.

Edwards, R., Temple, B. & Alexander, C. (2005). Users' experiences of interpreters: The critical role of trust. *Interpreting* 7 (1), 77–95.

Flores, G., Laws, M. B., Mayo, S. J., Zuckerman, B., Abreu, M., Medina, L. & Hardt, E. J. (2003). Errors in medical interpretation and their potential clinical consequences in pediatric encounters. *Pediatrics* 111 (1), 6–14.

Ginsberg, C., Martin, V., Andrulis, D., Shaw-Taylor, Y. & McGregor, C. (1995). *Interpretation and translation services in health care: A survey of US public and private teaching hospitals.* Washington, DC: National Public Health and Hospital Institute.

Jacobs, E. A., Agger-Gupta, N., Chen, A. H., Piotrowski, A. & Hardt, E. J. (2003). *Language barriers in health care settings: An annotated bibliography of the research literature.* Woodland Hills, CA: The California Endowment.

Kaufert, J. M. & Koolage, W. W. (1984). Role conflict among "culture brokers": The experience of native Canadian medical interpreters. *Social Science & Medicine* 18, 283–286.

Lang, R. (1975). Orderlies as interpreters in Papua New Guinea. *Papua New Guinea Medical Journal* 18 (3), 172–177.

Launer, J. (1978). Taking medical histories through interpreters: Practice in a Nigerian outpatient department. *British Medical Journal* 277, 934–935.

Metzger, M. (1999). *Sign language interpreting: Deconstructing the myth of neutrality.* Washington, DC: Gallaudet University Press.

Pöchhacker, F. (2000a). The community interpreter's task: Self-perception and provider views. In R. P. Roberts, S. E. Carr, D. Abraham & A. Dufour (Eds.), *The Critical Link 2: Interpreters in the community.* Amsterdam/Philadelphia, John Benjamins, 49–65.

Pöchhacker, F. (2000b). Language barriers in Vienna hospitals. *Ethnicity & Health* 5 (2), 113–119.

Pöchhacker, F. (2004). *Introducing interpreting studies.* London/New York: Routledge.

Pöchhacker, F. (2006). Research and methodology in healthcare interpreting. In E. Hertog & B. van der Veer (Eds.), *Taking stock: Research and methodology in community interpreting. Linguistica Antverpiensia, New Series,* 6, 135–159.

Price, J. (1975). Foreign language interpreting in psychiatric practice. *Australian and New Zealand Journal of Psychiatry* 9, 263–267.

Putsch, R. W. (1985). Cross-cultural communication: The special case of interpreters in health care. *Journal of the American Medical Association* 254 (23), 3344–3348.

Sarangi, S. (2004). Towards a communicative mentality in medical and healthcare practice. *Communication & Medicine* 1 (1), 1–11.

van Dijk, T. A. (Ed.) (1997). *Discourse as social interaction. Discourse studies: A multidisciplinary introduction,* vol. 2. London/Thousand Oaks/New Delhi: Sage.

Wadensjö, C. (1992). *Interpreting as interaction: On dialogue interpreting in immigration hearings and medical encounters.* Linköping: Linköping University Press.

Wadensjö, C. (1998). *Interpreting as interaction.* London/New York: Longman.

Wadensjö, C. (2001). Interpreting in crisis: The interpreter's position in therapeutic encounters. In I. Mason (Ed.), *Triadic exchanges. Studies in dialogue interpreting.* Manchester: St. Jerome, 71–85.

Woloshin, S., Bickell, N. A., Schwartz, L. M., Gany, F. & Welch, G. (1995). Language barriers in medicine in the United States. *Journal of the American Medical Association* 273 (9), 724–728.

Roles of community interpreters in pediatrics as seen by interpreters, physicians and researchers[1]

Yvan Leanza
University of Geneva & McGill University

This paper is an attempt at defining more clearly the various roles of community interpreters and the processes implicitly connected with each of them. While the role of the interpreter is a subject that has been widely discussed in the social science literature, it is less present in the biomedical one, which tends to emphasize the importance of interpreting in overcoming language barriers, rather than as a means of building bridges between patients and physicians. Hence, studies looking at interpreted medical interactions suggest that the presence of an interpreter is more beneficial to the healthcare providers than to the patient. This statement is illustrated by the results of a recent study in a pediatric outpatient clinic in Switzerland. It is suggested that, in the consultations, interpreters act mainly as linguistic agents and health system agents and rarely as community agents. This is consistent with the pediatricians' view of the interpreter as mainly a translating machine. A new typology of the varying roles of the interpreter is proposed, outlining the relation to cultural differences maintained therein. Some recommendations for the training of interpreters and healthcare providers are suggested.

Professionally interpreted consultations: A must for culturally sensitive health care

Language barriers in health care have been explored in many studies reported in the biomedical literature. There is strong evidence that the whole healthcare process is at risk when these barriers are not overcome. For example, language differences between patient and clinician are associated with inappropriate diagnostic investigations (Hampers et al. 1999), lower adherence to treatment (David & Rhee 1998; Karter et al. 2000; Manson 1988), lower rates of follow-up (appointments proposed and kept), poor referrals, incomplete investigations

(Sarver & Baker 2000) and lower rates of preventive interventions by physicians (Hu & Covell 1986; Solis et al. 1990; Woloshin et al. 1997). These difficult consultations place patients at risk for misdiagnosis, which can lead to inappropriate or inadequate treatment (Vasquez & Javier 1991) or to unnecessary hospital admissions (Hampers & McNulty 2002). Both patients (Carrasquillo et al. 1999; Morales et al. 1999) and healthcare providers (Leanza 2005; Raval & Smith 2003) may have a low rate of satisfaction in these situations.

One approach to addressing these barriers is to work with an interpreter. Studies suggest that interpreters employed in medical settings tend to be ad hoc or proxy interpreters, that is, untrained people drawn from the patient's family or the (non-medical) staff of the institution where the consultation takes place. While this strategy addresses the issue of language, it raises other important problems. There remain risks of misdiagnosis of patients (Vasquez & Javier 1991), and consultations are less likely to help the patient express difficult feelings or events (Eytan et al. 2002); confidentiality is not assured, and there is evidence that untrained interpreters feel significant stress and discomfort (Sasso 2000). When children interpret for their parents, not only are the dynamics of the family challenged (Ngo-Metzger et al. 2003), but the children themselves may be at severe risk for psychological sequels (Jacobs et al. 1995)[2].

It is evident that better medical care is obtained with the use of trained community[3] interpreters. If the goal is the best care possible, it is an ethical imperative to hire such professionals in medical settings (Blake 2003). But interpreting in medical settings is not only about "best practices"; it also involves larger social issues (i.e., the integration of minority or allophone groups into the society). Contrary to the frequently voiced concern that the use of interpreters will hamper the social and cultural integration of new immigrants, the provision of interpreting services involves acknowledging differences and diversity in what is usually a very normative institutional context. Integration, as opposed to assimilation, is a mutual adaptation process and also a joint process of meaning construction (Perregaux et al. 2001). It begins in the social institutions (schools, justice, welfare and health care), where interpreters may be crucial. Indeed, interpreters in these settings have many roles beyond being "translation machines"; they can facilitate intercultural communication, construct bridges between different symbolic universes and facilitate the process of migrant integration.

The biomedical literature rarely addresses these larger issues. For example Flores et al. (2002) underline the benefit of having a professional interpreter for pediatric care as this can permit the physician to obtain information about folk explanations and treatments. This information may help prevent harmful, even fatal, folk treatments. However, these authors make no mention of the role of the interpreter as a cultural mediator or an advocate for patients, improving their level of understanding of medical care and their feeling of being respectfully received and treated. In contrast to the narrow focus in the medical literature, work on interpreters' roles in social sciences ranges more widely (e.g. Cohen-Emerique 2003; Drennan & Swartz 1999; Jalbert 1998; Roberts 1997; Weiss & Stuker 1998) but remains mainly theoretical, with few empirical studies.

The first aim of this paper is to present some recent (mainly francophone) research done on "interpreted interaction" in medical settings, with an emphasis on interpreters' roles. This brief review will be followed by a presentation of some results from a study conducted at a pediatric outpatient clinic in Switzerland. The purpose of the study, anchored in a cross-cultural psychology framework and rooted in a complementarist epistemology (Devereux 1970), is to explore the kinds of relationship that healthcare professionals, in this case pediatricians, maintain with respect to cultural difference, and how the presence of interpreters affects this relationship. The theoretical framework (called the professional activities niche) not only emphasizes the individual experience, but also addresses the need to explore (1) the context where the professional activities take place (here a pediatric hospital and Swiss society); (2) the actual practice going on (here interpreted preventive pediatric consultations) and (3) the ethnotheories (or representations) of the healthcare professionals, i.e. the norms for being a good physician and for child rearing. In the study, interpreters' roles, viewed from the perspectives of the interpreters themselves, physicians, and the researcher, are considered as indicators of the processes going on in the construction of the relationship to the Other. The second aim of this paper is therefore to present the results with a focus on interpreters' roles. In other words, the broad question which will be addressed is: Do interpreters help building bridges between two symbolic worlds? The conclusion proposes a new typology for interpreters' roles that addresses the complex (and sometimes ambivalent) polyvalence of their work.

Communication facilitator or cultural assimilator?

Jalbert (1998) has proposed a useful typology, based primarily on the seminal work of the Winnipeg group (Kaufert 1990; Kaufert & Koolage 1984; Kaufert & Putsch 1997; Kaufert et al. 1998), to understand the varying roles of the interpreter:

1. *Translator*[4]: The interpreter minimizes her presence as much as possible. In this role she simply facilitates the communication process, not interfering with what the speakers say.

2. *Cultural Informant*: The interpreter helps the healthcare provider to better understand the patient. In this role the interpreter uses her knowledge of cultural norms and values.

3. *Culture Broker or Cultural Mediator*: The interpreter is a Cultural Informant but also a negotiator between two conflicting value systems or symbolic universes. In this role, the Culture Broker needs to enlarge, provide explanations or synthesize healthcare providers' and patients' utterances to help both parties arrive at a meaningful shared model (of care, of behavior etc.).

4. *Advocate*: In a value-conflict situation, the interpreter may choose to defend the patient against the institution.

5. *Bilingual Professional*: The interpreter becomes the healthcare professional. She leads the interview in the patient's language and then reports to the healthcare provider. She can do this because of prior training in health care or, in a more limited way, because of her knowledge of institutional practices and routines.

This typology has the advantage of not contrasting translation and mediation (or instrumental interpreting versus cultural mediation), which has often been the case in previous theorizing. French authors such as Cohen-Emerique (2003) or Delcroix (1996) tend to dichotomize interpreters' roles and by doing so, neglect the linguistic part of their work. This may obscure the potential assimilation power of their position; i.e. the possibility for the interpreter to be more a spokesperson for the institutional (dominant) discourse, a potential described by Davidson as the power "to keep the interview 'on track' and the physician on schedule" (2000:400).

In Jalbert's view, the Cultural Mediator's role appears only when there is a conflictual situation. In this case, the interpreter can contribute to conflict resolution. The typology also recognizes that the interpreter may act as a protector of patients, i.e., as an Advocate. In most cases, filling this role requires the interpreter to be well informed about the laws, rules and procedures that govern institutional practices. The interpreter may also be a Bilingual Professional, meaning that she is in essentially the same (symbolic) position as the healthcare provider. This implies that there is an agreement between the healthcare provider and the interpreter before the consultation starts. In a way, this role is the counterpart of the Advocate one, in that the interpreter is an agent of the institution and a spokesperson for the healthcare system and its discourse. Indeed, in the role of Bilingual Professional the interpreter may act in opposition to the cultural norms and values of her own community.

In the role of Translator, the interpreter attempts to be "invisible" and avoids any level of personal involvement. One can understand that in all roles but Translator, the interpreter is not expected to completely maintain the ideal of impartiality and must proceed on the basis of identifying either with the community (as Cultural Informant, Culture Broker and Advocate) or with the institution (Bilingual Professional). This is consistent with Bot's (2003) argument that "mythological neutrality" should be challenged based on the settings in which the interpreter works. It may be pertinent in legal settings, but not in medical or social settings, where personal involvement may be in the interest to both patient and care provider. Often, as in France (and now in Switzerland; see note 6), community interpreter codes of ethics are inspired by those of social mediators (such as family mediators or school mediators). Impartiality is thus a strong professional principle (see for example Bonafé-Schmitt et al. 1999, for social mediations in France). In community interpreting, as implied in Jalbert's theorizing, this impartiality is not possible nor even desirable. Not only is cultural knowledge needed, but experiences of migration and with the receiving country's institutions are necessary for professional community interpreting practice. This point challenges not only social mediation rules, but also the physician's "affective neutrality" which, according to Parsons' (1970) seminal work, is a key value for the medical profession.

Jalbert's typology describes idealized views of the various roles played by interpreters in medical settings. But what actually happens in interpreted healthcare consultations? Do interpreters' actions fall discretely into these categories? And, at the more basic level of the process of interpretation and mediation, how does the building of shared meaning take place?

Two studies reveal some of the complex roles and polyvalent actions of interpreters, who, usually hired as communication facilitators, implicitly become cultural assimilators. Traverso (2002), using qualitative linguistic analysis of exchanges between pregnant women, interpreters and healthcare providers in a French obstetrics and gynecology clinic, found that the interaction was more regular and fluid when an interpreter was present. But this third-party presence tended to exclude the patient from the interaction. The interpreter and the physician often talked about the mother and her pregnancy without speaking to her. The interpreter acted as a Professional. Not as a Bilingual Professional, as described by Jalbert (1998), but as a Monolingual healthcare Professional discussing the "case" with a colleague, here a gynecologist.

Grin (2003), an anthropologist, used participant observation to study interpreters' roles in different medical settings in French-speaking Switzerland. Her observations were part of a larger project examining the introduction of trained community interpreters in these institutions (Guex & Singy 2003). Many of these settings involved work with asylum seekers. In the first medical visit upon arriving in Switzerland, nurses had the administrative task of completing a medical file for each new asylum seeker. According to the nurses, this "written relation" to health care required a word-for-word translation of the patient's history. The main interpreter role was that of Translator. This emphasis on literal translation was not the case in an outpatient clinic, where the interpreters tended to play the role of Cultural Informants. The interpreters often added contextual details that helped the physician give a medical meaning to what had happened to the patient. Grin (2003) did not specify whether this cultural interpretation was one-way only or if it also involved giving the patient some contextual information for a better understanding of the medical discourse. In the obstetrics and gynecology clinics, where an interpreter was regularly present in follow-up visits by pregnant women, Grin found the interpreter playing the role of Bilingual Professional, acting almost autonomously. In this case, the physician and the interpreter had an agreement about the goals and procedure of the consultation. The interpreter conducted the interview in the patient's language and then reported the findings to the physician.

Grin also made some observations regarding a psychotherapeutic setting, in which interpreters were sometimes explicitly asked to be co-therapists: their involvement in the emotional work of therapy was considered crucial for patients' progress. In one case, Grin observed a therapist using an interpreter to do hypnosis. This observation is consistent with other research done in the psychotherapeutic milieu. The importance of the emotional and symbolic work done in psychotherapy may encourage a broadening of the interpreter's role to include a bridge-building process (Goguikian Ratcliff & Changkakoti 2004).

These studies make it clear that interpreters' roles differ widely from one context to another. Where there is an institutional need for cultural information or mediation, interpreters will be asked to perform these tasks, moving beyond their specific linguistic skills. But these studies have emphasized context-based analyses of the roles of interpreters and have not given attention to interpersonal factors — that is, to the quality and process of the relationship between the healthcare provider and the interpreter. Nor have they examined what happens in encounters where a value conflict appears or when the interpreter plays a role other than the one expected by the clinician (e.g., as Mediator or Advocate instead of Translator or Bilingual Professional). Many other interesting questions remain to be examined, including: How do different medical institutions create space for these new collaborators? What is their institutional status? Are they viewed as professionals in their own right or as a "tool" at hand, waiting to be used at the healthcare provider's will? Taken together, previous studies seem to suggest that in most settings involving medical interpreting, the institution's discourse remains the dominant one. The asymmetric relationship between patient and healthcare provider is rarely challenged by the presence of interpreters.

In summary, when researchers observe what happens in medical interactions involving an interpreter, they generally find that the dominant discourse of the institution is confirmed by the intervention of the interpreter (see also Bolden 2000; Davidson 2000; Wadensjö 1998). Where a shift in power and expression occurs, it reflects an institutional history and willingness to provide health care beyond the traditional biomedical standards, as was seen for example in Grin's observations for the psychotherapeutic setting. As pediatrics often defines itself as a specialization focused not only on the biomedical needs of the child but also on the psychosocial issues of child development and health, it is interesting to examine interpreting and cross-cultural issues in this particular context.

The "Education, pediatrics and culture" study

The study entitled "Education, pediatrics and culture" (Leanza 2003) was designed to examine not only interpreters' roles, but the whole experience of working with cultural differences in a pediatric setting, first from the perspective of the physicians and second from the interpreters' view, as they showed an interest in the research process. Methods included participant observation in a pediatric outpatient clinic in French-speaking Switzerland, videotaping of consultations for subsequent analysis of communication and the interpreter's role, and stimulated recall interviews with physicians and interpreters.

Preventive pediatrics

The pediatric consultations observed and analyzed were well-child visits, also called preventive consultations. In these encounters, the pediatrician not only explores the physical well-being of the child, but also monitors the psychosocial conditions of the child's development. She checks with the parents on how the child eats, sleeps and socializes. These topics, which are deeply rooted in cultures and psychosocial contexts, constitute the focus of interest in this study. As many cross-cultural developmental studies have shown, they are key factors in a child's enculturation and socialization (Dasen 2003). Preventive consultations should enable parents to pose questions and express concerns about their child's development. It is also a privileged opportunity to observe how psychosocial and cultural issues are dealt with in pediatrics. Before giving more details about the interpreters' roles in these encounters, I will briefly summarize the main results from the analyses of the context, of pediatricians' representations of their work, and of the child-rearing practices with which they were confronted.

Observations of the context revealed tensions between a willingness for change and an implicit desire to maintain the status quo. The highest levels of the hierarchy expressed their willingness to change how the institution dealt with these migrant populations. For example, this was expressed by the presence of interpreters and by monthly symposia for healthcare providers on "migration, cultures and care." But this willingness seemed to be in constant conflict with the operational realities of the hospital. For example, follow-up consultations were not necessarily performed by the same resident, and this lack of continuity was clearly counterproductive. Moreover, the resident's evaluation neglected the relational and socio-cultural dimensions of clinical practice. Thus, while there was a willingness to innovate, to make the whole pediatric practice more open to the subjectivity and social worlds of the patient, there was also inertia common to all institutions. The result was a tendency to break the very links that the practice innovations had attempted to create.

Two types of care providers' representations were examined: practice models, and norms relating to education that had to be transmitted to the families. These representations were not varied with respect to the diversity of the patient population. The procedure of the consultations inexorably followed the same sequence, whatever the parents' requests or the interpreters' interventions. Educational norms were also rigidly transmitted. For example, a chart describing the sequence for introducing solid food was distributed to the parents. This chart came from a pediatrics manual and was translated literally into Albanian and Tamil without any adaptation. It contained details of every meal measured to the gram, and implicitly suggested that breastfeeding was to be stopped at four months.

Communication analyses of these consultations revealed systematic interruptions, and apparent unawareness of socio-cultural dimensions of the child's development (Leanza 2004). The analyses of clinical practices and representations revealed that, despite the intention to develop a culturally responsive and innovative practice, pediatrics as practiced in this institution was quite conventional, in that it was not very patient-centric and excluded attention to socio-cultural and emotional factors.

Nevertheless, the clinic did provide interpreting services and I will examine some specific questions about the role of interpreters in pediatric consultations:

(1) How did pediatricians see interpreters' activities?
(2) How did interpreters see their own activities?
(3) Did the interpreter allow for or seek out cultural factors? What kind of interventions did the interpreter make?

The first and second questions are answered by using material from the stimulated recall interviews (as it is the experience of each participant which is sought) and the third by analyzing the actual role of interpreters in videotaped consultations (as it is the practice itself that is analyzed).

The pediatricians' view

Participants, data and methodology

The physicians participating in the study were eight pediatrics residents. Seven were female. All but one were training to become pediatricians; one was in a GP program completing the required residency in pediatrics. Participants had an average working experience of two years, except for the "GP resident," who was doing pediatrics for the first time. None of them had had any experience with such preventive consultations before starting their residency in this hospital. None had received any specific training in cross-cultural medicine or patient-physician relations.

One-on-one stimulated recall interviews based on the video recordings were conducted in the hospital. As the resident was watching herself (and only herself, not a colleague) doing a consultation, she was asked to react to what was representative for her about these preventive consultations with migrant families. At the same time, if the physician would not react to a phenomenon that was of importance to this study (such as an interpreter giving her opinion on a parental practice), I would introduce it by asking an open question (e.g., "What is it like to work with interpreters?"), orienting our dialogue toward these specific issues. On average, the interviews lasted between ninety minutes and two hours. They were transcribed and analyzed using N'Vivo 1 software (Nud*ist vivo 1998–1999), which supports content analysis (with preconceived and emerging categories) as well as theory building. The account of pediatricians' experience of working with cultural difference is presented in another paper (Leanza 2005). The results presented here are only a (consistent) fragment of the broader analysis, focusing on interpreters.

The interpreter as a "neutral ally"

Residents' comments about the videotaped consultations revealed two trends. The strongest one was to say that communication with parents and children was more difficult when an interpreter was present. These physicians found it very hard to get the information needed to do their work properly and manage time appropriately (according to institution rules). They felt a loss of control in their consultation and at times also felt excluded from the interaction with the parent. Pediatricians generally referred to the interpreter as a Translator, i.e., as "invisible," or as "allied" with the clinician, thus serving to get the biomedical message across to the parents. In residents' view, the interpreter may be a Cultural Informant, but only in the direction of physician to parent, and sometimes a Bilingual Professional, conveying the proper child nutrition instructions.

The second trend was much less pronounced than the first. It appeared in the comments of two residents. For these pediatricians, the contact with interpreters provided an opportunity to modify their representations of child rearing. They had tried to adapt their discourse to the reality and customs of the parents. In this perspective, the interpreter is not only a Translator or a medium for transmitting biomedical norms. The interpreter can also teach the professional something meaningful and thus serves as a two-way Cultural Informant. These pediatricians also see a "new" role for the interpreter, not noted in Jalbert's typology: they are aware that the interpreter has an important role outside the consultation room as a Support for the families. They mention the informal follow-up interpreters do in the community, for example by repeating explanations for prescriptions to the parents.

Neither Mediator nor Advocate roles are ever noted or acknowledged by the clinicians. They appear to see interpreters in the manner presupposed by the official code of ethics: as a neutral "translating machine" or neutral ally in the consultation. Such perceptions may well pose a challenge to the physician's position, ethics, knowledge and power. Overall, it seems that for the pediatrician, the interpreter is mainly an instrument for obtaining or transmitting information, and is only rarely seen as a real actor in the clinical interaction with whom beneficial collaboration may occur.

The interpreters' view

Participants, data and methodology

There were four interpreters involved in the study. Three of them were female and had been hired part-time by the hospital (two for Albanian patients and one for Tamil) four years earlier; the fourth was male and worked as a substitute for one of the Albanian-speaking interpreters. They were all from the cultural communities for which they interpreted and had a more or less difficult history of migration to Switzerland. All four had children (from newborn to adolescent). The three hired interpreters had received professional training from a local association, *Appartenances*. This training was based on three principles: (1) working on personal experiences; (2) interpreting techniques; and (3) knowledge about institutions (Métraux & Fleury 1997). It involved about 80 hours of classroom work, plus some supervised experience. The substitute interpreter had not received any training. Observed consultations were always interpreted by one of these four interpreters. Because of personal difficulties, only two interviews could be done, one with the Tamil interpreter and one with an Albanian interpreter, both trained as community interpreters.

The interviews were conducted in French, following the same procedure as the one followed with the pediatricians. The consultations or extracts of consultations shown to interpreters were the same as those shown to the physicians, provided that the interview partner was the interpreter of the consultation. Content analysis was performed with N'Vivo 1.

Ambivalences

The interviews with the interpreters identified two additional roles not included in Jalbert's typology. The first one was welcoming: the interpreters acted as "Welcomers" of patients to the hospital. According to the interpreters, their presence gave parents and patients confidence to face and navigate through this unfamiliar environment. As confirmed by participant observation, both parents and children felt more welcome in an institution that hired people from their own community and in this way showed some acknowledgement of their difference. Interpreters also performed the greeting rituals at the beginning of the clinical consultation. Often, the physician gave the patient a quick handshake and then just walked to her desk and opened the patient's file. Some parents waited to be invited to take a seat. This is when the interpreter played a welcoming role, making up for the lack of culturally appropriate greeting rituals. Interpreters also did this before the physician came in, when families were asked to wait in the consultation room.

The second role played by the interpreter was Family Support outside the hospital, as noted also by a few of the physicians. The two new roles indicate that community interpreters work toward social integration also before and after the consultation.

Interpreters felt that the Translator role was the one most frequently requested and enacted, but that was also the most frustrating role for them. They agreed that they sometimes served as Cultural Informants, but only in a "one-way" mode (from physician to patient). If they tried to work in the other direction (from patient to physician) they found they were unable to influence the physicians' discourse.

The role of the Bilingual Professional as described by Jalbert (1998) was used from time to time, principally when the consultation involved nutrition issues. The interpreters enjoyed this role which allowed them to experience a different symbolic position, closer to that of the physician than the migrant. This position was usually approved by the healthcare provider. One interpreter described this role as "reciting her poetry," particularly on the topic of nutrition. This metaphor informs us about the meaning of the activity for the interpreter. First, she knows what to say by heart; it can be understood as quite a mechanical activity proving her professional skill. On the other hand, reciting poetry can be seen as a very enjoyable activity, because of the beauty of the language (though this may hardly apply to biomedical specialized language) and because of the pleasure of expressing prestigious knowledge and making a good impression on others.

According to the interviews with both the pediatric residents and the interpreters, much more weight was given to the institutional discourse (biomedicine) than to that of the parents. Although interpreters were sometimes frustrated by not playing more of a Mediator role, they found some satisfaction in playing the role of Bilingual Professional, which allowed them to experience a status quite different from that of their fellow migrant patients (Weber & Molina 2003). Here we see some ambivalence in the interpreters' roles, as they claim to be Culture Brokers, but appear to very much enjoy the role of the cultural assimilator.

Analysis of the recordings: The perspective of the researcher

Data and methodology

As stated earlier, the study is rooted in a complementarist epistemology, which implies different views of the same object through complementary analytical lenses. It is a way of not only giving an account of the complexity of the object under study, but also achieving internal validity by triangulation of sources (here: participants' views and actual practice) and methods (here: interviews along with content analysis and observations along with role analysis) (Lincoln & Guba 1985: 305–307). From this perspective, 36 critical incidents, drawn from the 21 videotaped preventive consultations, were used for the analysis of interpreter roles. I considered a sequence of the consultation as a critical incident when the area under discussion was an educational topic such as nutrition or sleep. They were "critical" in the sense that they matched the study interest (discourses about educational issues in a multicultural pediatric setting).

The critical incidents were transcribed in standard orthography, as the goal of the analysis was to identify roles at a macro-level of discourse and not in the micro-linguistic details of the interaction. Thus the transcriptions look like theater dialogues allowing the researcher to explore the roles of the interpreter "character." Roles are defined by how the interpreter positioned herself symbolically toward the object of the medical intervention (child education topics). This positioning can be done in many different ways, which can be seen as more or less active (e.g., Translator being a passive[5] role as the interpreter does not add any personal opinion/knowledge to the interaction, and Advocate being an active one, as she will give her own personal opinion/knowledge about the migrant family situation). The interpreter could intervene about parenting practices and knowledge from a particular symbolic perspective, identifying either with the institution (the system perspective, e.g., Bilingual Professional) or with her community (the community perspective, e.g., Cultural Informant). As the initial focus of my study was on the pediatricians' experience, only the French portions of the interaction were transcribed and coded. Interpreters' utterances were coded according to Jalbert's role definitions. A particular coding instance could be a single sentence (or a part of it) or several turns, depending on whether the interpreter maintained a particular stance toward the educational issue.

I considered the interpreter as acting in the Translator role mainly when she converted speech directly from Albanian or Tamil into French, and waited for a reaction from the physician without engaging actively in a same-language dialogue. The other roles usually appeared when interpreter and physician spoke French among themselves — described by Davidson (2002) as an "optional same-language turn" between the interpreter and the interpretee in the interpreted discourse. Jalbert's typology was not always sufficient to account for the interpreter's stance. Therefore, I added two more roles.

Interpreters' polyvalence

I first noticed that the interpreter could also be an Active Translator, which means that, before interpreting anything, she actively engages the physician to clarify what is to be transmitted to the parent. Her questions are meant to help her understand minor points or linguistic details, but they do not address meanings of biomedical interventions or parental practices. In this sense, the interpreter maintains a passive stance regarding the object of the consultation (child education). This is illustrated by the following dialogue from a consultation for a one-year-old girl from Sri Lanka (I stands for interpreter, D for doctor/physician and P for parents; the utterance coded as Active Translator is in bold).

Extract 1

D: Maintenant ils peuvent commencer à lui donner du lait de vache... Je sais
    qu'à la Migros maintenant il y a des nouveaux
    *Now they can start to give her cow milk... I know that now at the Migros [a
    Swiss grocery store] there are new...* (hesitates)

I: **Nouveau? Du lait de vache?**
    New? Cow milk?

[...]

D: Oui, c'est des petits laits pour enfants à partir d'un mois. Je crois que c'est
    Milupa, mais c'est vendu à la Migros. Puis ça je pense que c'est bien pour
    commencer.
    *Yes, it's small milks for children from a month old. I believe it's Milupa [brand
    name for baby food], but it is sold at Migros. Then, I think it's good to start
    with.*

I: **A la Migros il y en a?**
    One finds them at the Migros?

D: Oui, à la Migros.
    Yes, at Migros.

[The interpreter finally translates to the parents]

The second new role, Monolingual Professional, occurred when the interpreter
displayed her knowledge about health matters in a very biomedical way. The same
applies to displays of her knowledge about migration issues. In this case, the community interpreter acted as an equal-status professional and expressed her view on
a particular aspect of the situation to the physician (as shown by Traverso 2002).
The example in Extract 2, taken from a consultation with a one-year-old boy from
Kosovo, illustrates this (the utterance coded as Monolingual Professional is in
bold).

Extract 2

P: [in Albanian]

I: Des fois il mange bien, des fois il mange moins bien. Des soupes... ils don-
    nent la soupe, les viandes que je prépare pour nous il mange.
    *Sometimes he eats well, sometimes less well. Soups... they give soup, meats that
    I prepare for us, he eats.*

D: Bon, insiste sur le fait qu'il faut pas qu'il boivent que du lait. Parce que s'ils
    le bourrent de lait, le reste il ne va pas vouloir manger. Puis maintenant à 1
    an, il faut qu'il mange de tout. Le lait est important mais pas aussi important
    qu'avant. Il faudrait pas qu'il boivent que ça.
    *Okay, insist on the fact that he shouldn't drink milk only. Because if they fill him
    up with milk, he is not going to want to eat the rest. Then, he is one year old now,
    he must eat everything. Milk is important, but not as important as before. He
    shouldn't be drinking only this.*

I: Je lui demande quelle sorte de viande elle lui donne ou bien combien de fois par semaine?
    Do I ask her what kind of meat she's giving him or how many times a week?
D: Oui... et puis tu lui avais donné à elle la feuille?
    Yes... and then did you give her the sheet [the chart of solid food introduction]?
I: Je me rappelle pas je vais lui demander.
    I don't remember I will ask her.
D: Si jamais tu lui donnes.
    If not give it to her.

Instead of translating directly what the physician just said, the interpreter engages her by asking a question. This question shows, first, that the interpreter possesses biomedical knowledge relating to the educational issue under discussion (nutrition), and second, that she would like to ask the mother more than what the physician is requesting, as would a healthcare professional needing information to make her own judgment. However, she asks the physician's permission before speaking with the mother. Here, the interpreter gains the physician's approval in this professional role, in the sense that he accepts her initiative and even asks her about the nutrition sheet, implying that it is the interpreter's responsibility to make sure parents get this information (which is not the case according to hospital rules).

Sometimes the interpreter does not wait for the physician's approval to give her "professional opinion" on an educational topic, as illustrated in Extract 3 from the transcript of a consultation with the parents of an 18-month-old Albanian boy. The family was refused asylum in Switzerland and had only a few days left before leaving for Kosovo. At this time the mother asks some questions about the attendant consequences for her child's health:

Extract 3
[After a relatively long discussion between I and P in Albanian]
I: Elle pense qu'on va lui donner des vaccins pour le climat, le changement de climat. **Ça je lui ai dit non ça n'existe pas de ça, mais on va lui donner des vaccins...**
    She thinks that we will give him vaccines for the climate, for the climate change. This I told her no [D approves with a head nod] this does not exist, but we will give him vaccines...
D: Contre les maladies d'enfant.
    Against childhood diseases.

In this brief exchange one learns that the interpreter has already given her "medical" opinion to the mother. This is confirmed by the physician, first by her head nod and then by completing the interpreter's sentence before she can finish it herself. The interpreter puts herself in the position of a Bilingual Professional (in bold in the excerpt). In doing so, she interrupts the mother's request even before it is transmitted to the physician, which is slightly different from the previous role (Monolingual Professional), but the symbolic identification stays the same: the interpreter is positioning herself as a healthcare representative.

Another phenomenon is that of the interpreter choosing to give the physician information about the parents' practices, this time positioning herself as a community agent. She is then acting as a Cultural Informant, as shown in Extract 4, involving a nine-month-old Albanian boy (the utterance coded as Cultural Informant is in bold).

> **Extract 4**
> P: [in Albanian]
> I: La maman dit : la journée il tète très peu et il boit que les jus de fruit et c'est la nuit qu'il tète tout le temps.
> [With a big smile] *The mother says: during the day he nurses very little, and he only drinks fruit juices, and it's only at night that he nurses all the time.*
> D: Alors, moi je commencerai par arrêter de lui donner la tétée. Première chose il faut faire ça ! Puis après essayer de lui donner un horaire, puis quand il aura faim, il mangera. C'est que là il a pas faim.
> [After a disappointed gesture and a complicit smile to I] *So, I would start by stopping to nurse him. That's the first thing to do! Then try to get him on a schedule, then when he will be hungry, he will eat. The problem is he is not hungry.*
> I-P [Exchange in Albanian]
> I: Elle a l'impression qu'elle n'a pas assez de lait.
> *She has the impression that she does not have enough milk.*
> D: Mais ça ne m'étonne pas !
> *But that doesn't surprise me!*
> I: Et c'est pour ça, elle dit, je… le garde toute… la nuit au sein.
> *And that's why, she says, I… keep him all… night long at my breast.*
> D   (sigh)
> I: **Tu sais chez nous y a pas d'horaire. Tous les… le jour, la nuit…**
> *You know with us there is no schedule. All… day, night…*
> D: Je sais.
> *I know.*
> I: **La nuit même c'est même pas compté, hein. Si on lui demande s'il mange la nuit et ils répondent que la journée…**
> *Even night is not even taken into account, hm. If one asks her if he eats at night and they answer only about the day…*
> [Someone from administration comes into the consultation room, interrupting the dialogue. I walks out to interpret for someone else. When she comes back, nutrition is not addressed any more].

Information transmitted here to the physician (the practice of breastfeeding at night) does not change at all the standard prescription that the healthcare provider gives to the parent (stop breastfeeding as the child is already 9 months old and give him a nutrition schedule). The physician says she is already aware of this parental practice, but this awareness does not seem to help her take some distance from the biomedical norms. Certainly, there may be a real nutrition problem, given that the child does not seem to consume anything other than fruit juices and breast milk. However, the child's development was assessed as completely normal. Throughout, the physician remains in the position of an expert trying to correct the deficient knowledge base of the parents. She does not enter into a negotiation process, or, with interpreter's help, try to understand the parents' perspective and so identify a strategy to help the mother change her nutritional practices.

Quantified results: The dominant stays dominant

The results of the coding of all the critical incidents are shown in Figure 1. Out of 187 interpreters' utterances, 167 (i.e. roughly 90%) were in one of the two Translator roles. The remaining 20 utterances (i.e. roughly 10%) were distributed among

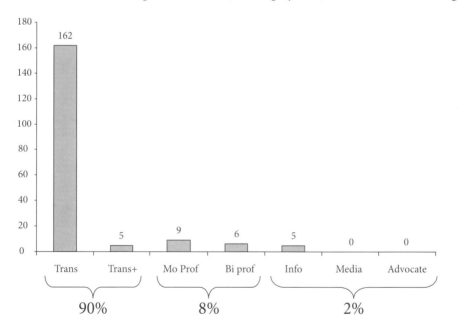

Figure 1. Number of coding instances of interpreters' roles in sequences about education topics

Note: Trans = Translator; Trans+ = Active Translator; Mo Prof = Monolingual Professional; Bi Prof = Bilingual Professional; Info = Cultural Informant; Media = Cultural Mediator

Bilingual Professional, Monolingual Professional and Cultural Informant. In the sequences analyzed, the interpreters never played the Mediator or Advocate roles.

These quantified results are consistent not only with the physicians' and interpreters' points of view, as expressed in the research interviews, but also with the interpreters' code of ethics[6], which emphasizes "neutrality." It appears then that this "neutrality" is based on the tacit agreement between the interpreter, on the one hand, and the professional and the institution, on the other — and it serves the dominant discourse. The main task that physicians expected from the interpreters was translation, and sometimes the transmission of biomedical norms about educational topics. That is what the interpreters felt they were doing, even if they found it frustrating, and systematic observation indicates that this was what indeed happened in the consultations.

The actual proportion of utterances in the critical passages that were spent in translation as opposed to more personal and active interventions (90% versus 10%) is to be expected, given that the interpreter is in the consultation room first to overcome the language barrier. What is more surprising is the considerable proportion (8%) of utterances as health system agent, compared to only 2% as Cultural Informant. Evidently, the only roles the interpreter can play outside the health-related ones are those that do not pose a challenge to the physicians' power and position. This means, however, that interpreters are not able to help build a two-way bridge of communication between the physician and patient.

This failure to build a full partnership can be explained by three factors. First, the pediatric residents were not trained to work with interpreters. Some of them were not even aware of the different skills a community interpreter has, such as being able to give some information about cultural practices and values. Two of the physicians only became aware of this during the research interview when they were asked where they could find information about a particular practice. In a way, clinicians were inclined toward a mechanical effort to get the information across rather than engage in negotiation or broader discussion, because they lacked confidence and wanted to achieve a basic level of competence, narrowly defined by their perception of their own role as trainees. Second, the interpreters are not trained to be assertive in the face of institutional authority. For example, the Advocate role was not addressed in their training. As stated, they had an ambiguous relationship with medicine, which allowed them to temporarily experience a higher status than that of their fellow countrymen. Third, the whole outpatient-clinic context is struggling to introduce effective changes in clinical routines. However, this is not clearly supportive of practicing a more socio-culturally oriented pediatrics. The assimilative process going on in the consultation (and institution) is consistent with the non-participative assimilationist socio-cultural insertion which Switzerland "offers" to migrants (Bolzman 2001).

Conclusion: A new typology of roles and recommendations for training

Based on my empirical findings, I propose a synthesis and new organization of interpreters' roles. Each of the squares in Figure 2 is a particular way of approaching cultural difference for the community interpreter:

- As a *system agent,* the interpreter transmits the dominant discourse, norms and values to the patient. Cultural difference is denied in favor of the dominant culture. Cultural difference tends to be elided or assimilated.
- As a *community agent,* the interpreter plays the reverse role: the minority (migrant) norms and values are presented as potentially equally valid. Cultural difference is acknowledged. This role can be played in various ways, more or less nuanced.
- When acting as an *integration agent*, the interpreter finds resources to help migrants (and people from the receiving society) to make sense, negotiate meanings and find an "in-between" way of behaving. These roles take place outside consultations in everyday life.
- As a *linguistic agent*, the interpreter attempts to maintain an impartial position (to the extent that this is possible). The relationship with cultural difference is more technical, in that the interpreter has to find the proper translation on the fly. The cognitive and symbolic process does not require her to intervene on any level other than that of language (in other words, she does not intervene about the object of the interaction).

This study has implications for the training of interpreters. The future interpreter should explore all these potential roles during her training. Professionalization of interpreters must consider the ethical and pragmatic dimensions of these different roles and their implications for institutions, clients, and the interpreters themselves. The temptation for interpreters to differentiate themselves from their fellow countrymen by asserting their symbolic biomedical position should be challenged

System agent Bilingual Professional Monolingual Professional	Integration agent Welcoming Support - Follow up
Community interpreter	
Community agent Cultural Informant Culture Broker Advocate	Linguistic agent Translator (±Active)

Figure 2. Community interpreter's roles according to their relation to cultural difference

by giving them an official status distinct from that of the healthcare provider, acknowledged as professionals in their own right. One way to do this would be to give more autonomy to interpreters for this kind of work. This would also help contain the assimilative discourse and prevent it from being extended to all medical activity.

The study also points to the need for training healthcare providers (as well as other professionals) to work with interpreters. Although this would seem quite basic, in Switzerland at least there is either no training at all (in the majority of programs), or else exposure to a very technical set of guidelines (Bischoff & Loutan 1998). These guidelines concern what the professional should do before, during and after the interaction, and what he should not do. While this is a necessary framework, it is not sufficient. The interpreters' work is not only "passive" translation, which is usually implicit in this kind of technical training; it also involves active symbolic, affective and interactional dimensions which need to be understood as such by healthcare providers. These aspects of working with interpreters cannot be taught as a list of dos and don'ts.

Professional training for working with interpreters requires a follow-up in healthcare institutions, for example by setting up of what the French educational scientist Bourgeois (1996) calls a "safe training space," where professional identity can adapt to a new and challenging activity. This space must be one in which the medical professional's anxiety over losing control of the process and his/her feeling that "I won't get the right information to make a proper diagnostic" can be acknowledged without jeopardizing his/her evaluation. Such openness will in fact encourage the honing of skills and the consolidation of professional identity. This is a challenge for young professionals, as they have to negotiate the complexity and uncertainty of working with interpreters with their efforts to acquire basic skills and expertise.

This study also identifies needs for further research. First, knowledge about interpreters' roles outside the institutions — that is, in the community, when they endorse the (almost unnoticed) *integration agent* roles — may be of interest in trying to capture the whole complexity of the interpreters' position in a multicultural society. Second, there is a need for more data-driven studies on what happens in interpreted interactions, and in particular on the roles interpreters play in specific contexts, and with what implications. This would include studies similar to the one presented here, conducted with experienced physicians with the aim of establishing whether their views of the interpreter's role(s) as *system agent* and as *community agent* are suitably balanced. Such analyses should also be extended to other socio-medical contexts, so as to permit comparisons and the identification of setting-specific relationships, like those seen in psychiatry or psychotherapy.

Notes

1. I am grateful to Laurence J. Kirmayer, Ellen Rosenberg, Kelly McKinney and Steven Cohen for their comments on the first draft of this paper and their linguistic help. I also thank Margalit Cohen-Emerique for her insightful comments on my work, and Melissa Dominicé Dao for our discussions on the topic and her bibliographic help. And a special thanks to the two anonymous reviewers who gave me very precise and constructive comments.

2. This "pathologizing" view of children interpreting has recently been challenged by the results of very interesting research (Green et al. 2005).

3. "In the most general sense, community interpreting refers to interpreting in institutional settings of a given society in which public service providers and individual clients do not speak the same language" (Pöchhacker 1999: 126). It is often opposed to "conference interpreting" (simultaneous interpreting) and sometimes compared to sign language interpreting as sign interpreters follow their clients in different institutional settings. Community interpreting does not refer to a universally standardized practice as many factors (such as politics and economics) shape this activity from one region to another. Sometimes, the community interpreter can hold a university degree, while at other times she will have received only 6 hours of training or none at all (see Pöchhacker 1999).

4. To differentiate this particular role and the whole interpreting practice, I keep the "translator" term, being aware it is not the best term because there is translation in each role and because this is the usual way to name people who do written translations.

5. The term passive does not imply that the interpreter is an "automatic translating machine" or a "conduit." The use of this term is meant to qualify only the symbolic position, not all of the activities taking place, which, of course, implies numerous active processes, particularly at a cognitive and interactional level, as has been shown by many authors such as Angelelli (2000), Bélanger (2003), Davidson (2002) or Wadensjö (1998).

6. As of 4 June 2005, Swiss community interpreters do have a professional code. It was adopted at the general assembly of the INTERPRET' association. In this code, neutrality is defined as an obligation as is interpreters' contribution to "equality of chances and integration of migrants in a pluralistic society." These two statements can be seen as contradictory: how can one be neutral and at the same time promote integration (not assimilation)?

References

Angelelli, C. (2000). Interpretation as a communicative event: A look through Hymes' lenses. *Meta* 45 (4), 580–592.

Bélanger, D.-C. (2003). Les différentes figures d'interaction en interprétation de dialogue. In L. Brunette, G. Bastin, I. Hemlin & H. Clarke (Eds.), *The critical link 3*. Amsterdam/Philadelphia: John Benjamins, 51–66.

Bischoff, A. & Loutan, L. (1998). *A mots ouverts. Guide de l'entretien médical bilingue à l'usage des soignants et des interprètes*. Genève: Hôpitaux Universitaires de Genève.

Blake, C. (2003). Ethical considerations in working with culturally diverse populations: The essential role of professional interpreters. *Bulletin de l'association des psychiatres du Canada*, 6/2003, 21–23.

Bolden, G. (2000). Toward understanding practices of medical interpreting: Interpreters' involvement in history taking. *Discourse Studies* 2 (4), 387–419.

Bolzman, C. (2001). Quels droits citoyens? Une typologie des modèles d'intégration des migrants aux sociétés de résidence. In C. Perregaux, T. Ogay, Y. Leanza & P. Dasen (Eds.), *Intégrations et migrations. Regards pluridisciplinaires*. Paris: L'Harmattan, 159–183.

Bonafé-Schmitt, J.-P., Dahan, J., Salzer, J., Souquet, M. & Vouche, J.-P. (1999). *Les médiations, la médiation*. Ramonville Saint-Agne: Erès.

Bot, H. (2003). The myth of the uninvolved interpreter interpreting in mental health and the development of a three-person psychology. In L. Brunette, G. Bastin, I. Hemlin & H. Clarke (Eds.), *The critical link 3*. Amsterdam/Philadelphia: John Benjamins, 27–35.

Bourgeois, E. (1996). Identité et apprentissage. *Education permanente* 128, 27–35.

Carrasquillo, O., Orav, E., Brennan, T. & Burstin, H. (1999). Impact of language barriers on patient satisfaction in an emergency department. *Journal of General Internal Medicine* 14 (2), 82–87.

Cohen-Emerique, M. (2003). La médiation interculturelle, les médiateurs et leur formation. In F. Remotti (Ed.), *Corpi, individuali e contesti interculturali*. Turin: L'Harmattan Italia Connessioni, 58–87.

Dasen, P. (2003). Theoretical frameworks in cross-cultural developmental psychology: An attempt at integration. In T. Saraswathi (Ed.), *Cross-cultural perspectives in human development. Theory, research and applications*. New Dehli: Sage, 128–165.

David, R. & Rhee, M. (1998). The impact of language as a barrier to effective health care in an underserved urban Hispanic community. *Mount Sinai Journal of Medicine* 65 (5/6), 393–397.

Davidson, B. (2000). The interpreter as institutional gatekeeper: The social-linguistic role of interpreters in Spanish-English medical discourse. *Journal of Sociolinguistics* 4 (3), 379–405.

Davidson, B. (2002). A model for the construction of conversational common ground in interpreted discourse. *Journal of Pragmatics* 34, 1273–1300.

Delcroix, C. (1996). Rôles joués par les médiatrices socio-culturelles au sein du développement local et urbain. *Espaces et sociétés* 84–85, 153–176.

Devereux, G. (1970). *Essai d'ethnopsychiatrie générale*. Paris: Gallimard.

Drennan, G. & Swartz, L. (1999). A concept over-burdened: Institutional roles for psychiatric interpreters in post-apartheid South-Africa. *Interpreting* 4 (2), 169–198.

Eytan, A., Bischoff, A., Rrustemi, I., Durieux, S., Loutan, L., Gilbert, M., et al. (2002). Screening of mental disorders in asylum-seekers from Kosovo. *Australian and New Zealand Journal of Psychiatry* 36 (4), 499–503.

Flores, G., Rabke-Verani, J., Pine, W. & Sabharwal, A. (2002). The importance of cultural and linguistic issues in the emergency care of children. *Pediatric Emergency Care* 18 (4), 271–284.

Goguikian Ratcliff, B. & Changkakoti, N. (2004). Le rôle de l'interprète dans la construction de l'interculturalité dans un entretien ethnopsychiatrique. *L'autre. Cliniques, cultures et sociétés* 5 (2), 255–264.

Green, J., Free, C., Bhavnani, V. & Newman, A. (2005). Translators and mediators: Bilingual young people's accounts of their interpreting work in health care. *Social Science & Medicine* 60, 2097–2110.

Grin, C. (2003). Retour à la pratique. In P. Guex & P. Singy (Eds.), *Quand la médecine à besoin d'interprètes*. Genève: Médecine & Hygiène, 141–163.

Guex, P. & Singy, P. (Eds.) (2003). *Quand la médecine à besoin d'interprètes*. Genève: Médecine & Hygiène.

Hampers, L., Cha, S., Gutglass, D., Binns, H. & Krug, S. (1999). Language barriers and resource utilization in a pediatric emergency department. *Pediatrics* 103, 1253–1256.

Hampers, L. & McNulty, J. (2002). Professional interpreters and bilingual physicians in a pediatric emergency department: Effect on resource utilization. *Archives of Pediatrics & Adolescent Medicine* 156 (11), 1108–1113.

Hu, D. & Covell, R. (1986). Health care usage by Hispanic outpatients as function of primary language. *Western Journal of Medicine* 144 (4), 490–493.

Jacobs, B., Kroll, L., Green, J. & David, T. (1995). The hazards of using a child as an interpreter. *Journal of the Royal Society of Medicine* 88 (8), 474P–475P.

Jalbert, M. (1998). Travailler avec un interprète en consultation psychiatrique. *P.R.I.S.M.E.* 8 (3), 94–111.

Karter, A., Ferrara, A., Darbinian, J., Ackerson, L. & Selby, J. (2000). Self-monitoring of blood glucose: Language and financial barriers in a managed care population with diabetes. *Diabetes Care* 23 (4), 477–483.

Kaufert, J. (1990). Sociological and anthropological perpectives on the impact of interpreters on clinician/client communication. *Santé Culture Health* 7 (2/3), 209–235.

Kaufert, J. & Koolage, W. (1984). Role conflict among 'culture brokers': The experience of native Canadian medical interpreters. *Social Science & Medicine* 18 (3), 283–286.

Kaufert, J. & Putsch, R. (1997). Communication through interpreters in healthcare: Ethical dilemmas arising from differences in class, culture, language, and power. *Journal of Clinical Ethics* 8 (1), 71–87.

Kaufert, J., Putsch, R. & Lavallee, M. (1998). Experience of aboriginal health interpreters in mediation of conflicting values in end-of-life decision making. *International Journal of Circumpolar Health* 57, Suppl 1, 43–48.

Leanza, Y. (2003). *Education, pédiatrie et cultures. Du sens de l'activité professionnelle pour des pédiatres dans leur travail de prévention auprès de familles migrantes*. Unpublished doctoral dissertation, University of Geneva.

Leanza, Y. (2004). Pédiatres, parents migrants et interprètes communautaires: Un dialogue de sourds? *Cahiers de l'institut de linguistique et des sciences du langages (ILSL)* 16, 131–158.

Leanza, Y. (2005). Le rapport à l'autre culturel en milieu médical. L'exemple de consultations pédiatriques de prévention pour des familles migrantes. *Bulletin de l'Association pour la Recherche InterCulturelle* 41, 8–27.

Lincoln, Y. & Guba, E. (1985). *Naturalistic inquiry*. Beverly Hills: Sage.

Manson, A. (1988). Language concordance as a determinant of patient compliance and emergency room use in patients with asthma. *Medical Care* 26, 1119–1128.

Métraux, J.-C. & Fleury, F. (1997). La création du futur. La promotion de la santé dans des communautés migrantes et/ou affectées par la guerre. *Politiques sociales* 56 (1/2), 98–111.

Morales, L., Cunningham, W., Brown, J., Liu, H. & Hays, R. (1999). Are Latinos less satisfied with communication by health care providers? *Journal of General Internal Medicine* 14 (7), 409–417.

Ngo-Metzger, Q., Massagli, M., Clarridge, B., Manocchia, M., Davis, R., Iezzoni, L., et al. (2003). Linguistic and cultural barriers to care. *Journal of General Internal Medicine* 18 (1), 44–52.

Nud*ist (non-numerical unstructured data indexing, searching and theorizing) vivo (1998–1999). [software]. Victoria: Qualitative Solutions and Research (QSR).

Parsons, T. (1970). Structure sociale et procesus dynamique: Le cas de la pratique médicale moderne. In C. Herzlich (Ed.), *Medecine, maladie et societe*. Paris: Mouton.

Perregaux, C., Ogay, T., Leanza, Y. & Dasen, P. (Eds.). (2001). *Intégrations et migrations. Regards pluridisciplinaires*. Paris: L'Harmattan.

Pöchhacker, F. (1999). "Getting organized": The evolution of community interpreting. *Interpreting* 4 (1), 125–140.

Raval, H. & Smith, J. (2003). Therapists' experiences of working with language interpreters. *International Journal of Mental Health* 32 (2), 6–31.

Roberts, R. (1997). Community interpreting today and tomorrow. In S. E. Carr, R. Roberts, A. Dufour & D. Steyn (Eds.), *The critical link: Interpreters in the community*. Amsterdam/ Philadelphia: John Benjamins, 7–26.

Sarver, J. & Baker, D. (2000). Effect of language barriers on follow-up appointments after an emergency department visit. *Journal of General Internal Medicine* 15 (4), 256–264.

Sasso, A. (2000). *Interpreter services in health care: A call for provincial standards and services*. Vancouver: Affiliation of multicultural services agencies and societies of British Columbia.

Solis, J., Marks, G., Garcia, M. & Shelton, D. (1990). Acculturation, access to care, and use of preventive services by Hispanics: Findings from HHANES 1982–84. *American Journal of Public Health* 80 Suppl, 11–19.

Traverso, V. (2002). Rencontre interculturelle à l'hôpital: La consultation médicale avec interprète. *Travaux neuchatelois de linguistique* 36, 81–100.

Vasquez, C. & Javier, R. A. (1991). The problem with interpreters: Communicating with Spanish-speaking patients. *Hospital and Community Psychiatry* 42 (2), 163–165.

Wadensjö, C. (1998). *Interpreting as interaction*. London/New York: Longman.

Weber, O. & Molina, M. (2003). Le point de vue des médiateurs culturels/interprètes. In P. Guex & P. Singy (Eds.), *Quand la médecine à besoin d'interprètes*. Genève: Médecine & Hygiène, 85–112.

Weiss, R. & Stuker, R. (1998). *Interprétariat et médiation culturelle dans le système de soins* (Rapport no. 11). Neuchâtel: Forum Suisse pour l'Etude des Migrations.

Woloshin, S., Schwartz, L. M., Katz, S. J. & Welch, H. G. (1997). Is language a barrier to the use of preventive services? *Journal of General Internal Medicine* 12 (8), 472–477.

Doctor–patient consultations in dyadic and triadic exchanges[1]

Carmen Valero Garcés
University of Alcalá

This article presents the results of a study on doctor–patient interaction in dyadic and triadic exchanges. The analysis is based on transcripts of recordings done at healthcare centres in northern Madrid, Spain, and Minneapolis, USA. The methodological approach is that of institutional discourse analysis as developed by Drew and Heritage (Drew & Heritage 1992; Heritage 1995, 1997; Drew & Sorjonen 1997). Three different types of doctor–patient interaction are examined: (1) doctor/foreign-language patient; (2) doctor/ foreign-language patient/ad hoc interpreter; (3) doctor/ foreign-language patient/trained interpreter. Topics such as the assignment of participant roles, changes in the general structure, turn-taking, and asymmetrical relationships are explored. The study is mainly descriptive and qualitative, but also includes some comparative quantitative analyses.

1. Introduction

This paper sheds light on some salient features of cross-cultural doctor–patient interaction in three configurations: Type 1: doctor/foreign-language patient; Type 2: doctor/ foreign-language patient/ad hoc interpreter; and Type 3: doctor/ foreign-language patient/trained interpreter. The theoretical and methodological framework used (see Section 3.1) is that of institutional discourse analysis as developed by Drew and Heritage (Drew & Heritage 1992; Drew & Sorjonen 1997; Heritage 1995, 1997). Inspired by the work of Wadensjö (1992) and related discourse-analytical approaches (e.g. Mason 2001; Davidson 2002; Meyer 2001; Meyer et al. 2003), this study follows previous analyses of monolingual interactions between doctors and immigrant patients (Valero Garcés 2001, 2002, 2003). The article offers a comparative analysis of dyadic (monolingual) and triadic (bilingual interpreter-mediated) exchanges in doctor–patient interaction. The approach is primarily descriptive and qualitative, but also includes some quantification.

2. Corpus

The data in the study described below comes from six recordings made in hospitals and healthcare centres in northern Madrid, Spain (Type 1 and Type 2), and in Minneapolis, USA (Type 3). The data from Spain are part of the corpus of medical interviews collected by the FITISPos[2] research group at the University of Alcalá. The corpus is currently made up of 60 audiotaped monolingual and multilingual medical consultations of Type 1 and Type 2 recorded in healthcare centres, primarily in the departments of pediatrics, obstetrics, gynaecology and internal medicine and in the emergency room. Languages in the corpus include Arabic, Bulgarian, Polish, Portuguese and Romanian as well as Spanish. The participants are Spanish-speaking doctors and nurses, immigrant patients with some or practically no command of Spanish, and bilingual relatives of the patients, acting as ad hoc interpreters.

The Type-3 consultations were audiotaped at a hospital in Minneapolis and belong to a research group coordinated by Bruce Downing at the University of Minnesota, of which the author is a member. The Type-3 consultations from Minnesota were used for lack of such data in the Spanish corpus, since there are as yet few, if any, professional hospital interpreters in Spain. The interpreter involved in both Type-3 consultations had received two semesters of formal training at the University of Minnesota and had been working as an interpreter in a hospital for two years.

The consultations analysed in this paper are numbered from C1 to C6, and their main features (languages, participants, place, complaint) can be summarised as follows:

Type 1 — doctor/ foreign-language patient
C1 (Spanish): general practitioner (male) — Bulgarian patient (male) who knows some Spanish; healthcare centre in Guadalajara; leg problems.
C2 (Spanish): general practitioner (male) — Arabic-speaking patient (female) who knows some Spanish; healthcare centre in Alcalá de Henares; stomach problems.

Type 2 — doctor/foreign-language patient/ad hoc interpreter
C3 (Spanish-Arabic): general practitioner (male) — Moroccan patient (female) who does not speak Spanish — patient's husband acting as ad hoc interpreter; healthcare centre in Alcalá de Henares; stomach pains.
C4 (Spanish-Arabic): general practitioner (male) — Moroccan patient (female) who does not speak Spanish — patient's husband acting as ad hoc interpreter; healthcare centre in Alcalá de Henares; neck and back pains.

Type 3 — doctor/ foreign-language patient/trained interpreter

C5 (English-Spanish): specialist doctor (female) – Mexican patient (female) who does not speak English — interpreter (female) at a hospital in Minneapolis; vaginal infection.

C6 (English-Spanish): general practitioner (female) — Latino patient (female) who does not speak English — interpreter (female, same as in C5) at a hospital in Minneapolis; depression.

3. Analysis

3.1 Methodological framework

Research on institutional discourse shows that participants in institutional encounters use a series of linguistic and interactional resources specific to the situation, and in accordance with the participants' linguistic and cultural competencies. Many of these resources are also used in everyday conversation and are not exclusive to institutional encounters; they are, however, used in a specific way.

These resources are based on the following assumptions:

1. The participants have specific roles;
2. Each institutional context imposes certain constraints;
3. Each institution has its particular inference markers and its particular procedures.

According to Heritage (1997: 164), these assumptions are manifested in conversation through the use of linguistic and extralinguistic resources such as specific grammatical structures, turn exchanges, lexical choices and body language. The nonconventional or 'unexpected' use of these resources may change the assignment of participant roles, problems in understanding the intended meaning, and variation in the nature of relations with the institution as well as in the type of contribution. In the following sections these aspects of the three types of doctor–patient consultations described above will be analysed with the aim of investigating similarities and differences in the use of language.

3.2 Changes in the assignment of participant roles

The specific roles assigned to participants in doctor–patient encounters are similar to those seen in other interactions involving a professional-client relationship. The imbalance between the two parties is not an exception to the rule, but is intrinsic to the institutional context. If this system is altered, variation in the client's participation (Heritage 1997: 165) may result, including changes in the interaction order, the contribution types and the participants' expectations. These changes are all the more pronounced when one of the participants — the patient in our case — does not know the official language and the patterns of institutional organization. In such cases, processes of accommodation will take place, as shown in previous studies (Valero Garcés 2002).

Data from the present corpus also shows some changes in the use of Spanish in monolingual consultations (Type 1): the non-native-speaker patient speaks broken Spanish and takes on a more active role, e.g. by asking more questions or introducing topics that are not necessarily related to his/her illness. These may include documents or administrative procedures, such as appointments, as illustrated in Excerpt 1 (from C1):

> **Excerpt 1**[3]
> The doctor (D) wants to know when the patient (P) will be going to another hospital for an appointment.
>
> 10   D: Y aquí pondrían 1003… ¿Cuándo tienes que ir a la consulta?
> *And here it would say 1003 … When do you have to go to the appointment?*
>
> 11   P: ¿Cuál día?
> *Which day?*
>
> 12   D: Sí
> *Yes*
>
> 13   P: Yo primero hablar con jefe… Cuando descanso un día… Es que tu escribir un día… ¿puedo así?
> *Me first speak with boss … When I rest one day … when you write one day … can I do like that?*
>
> 14   D: Es que… yo te puedo citar para verte yo… um.. Yo puedo decir cuando vienes tú aquí… pero no cuando vas tú al hospital. Eso tiene que ser hospital quien dice cuando vas ¿vale?
> *The thing is that … I can make an appointment to see you … um … I can say when you come here … but not when you go to the hospital. It is hospital that says when you go. Okay?*
>
> 15   P: Sí, sí
> *Yes, yes.*

In this example, the patient speaks in broken Spanish and the doctor uses simplified structures. Specifically, we see that the patient needs clarification and asks a question (13) instead of answering the question asked by the doctor. The patient fails to respond because he lacks knowledge of the institutional reality, and it is the doctor who can provide him with the required information.

In Type-2 encounters, the ad hoc interpreter also takes this active role. He is the one who asks the doctor questions, makes comments, adds information or even omits it, as seen in Excerpt 2 (from C3):

Excerpt 2

The patient complains of stomachache and pain after eating. She has had thyroid surgery. Her husband, acting as ad hoc interpreter, is telling the doctor where his wife feels pain.

51 I: Le molesta aquí y por eso no puede ni vomitar ni nada, aquí
It bothers her here and for that reason she can neither vomit nor anything, here

52 P: (????) bocio
(????) goitre

53 I: Dice a ver si va ser el bocio, el bocio imposible porque ya te han quitado (????) el tiroides
She says it must be the goitre; it can't be the goitre because they have already taken out (????) the thyroid

54 D: Dile que el bocio es un aumento del tamaño del tiroides, que es una glándula
Tell him that the goitre is an increase of the size of the thyroid, which is a gland

55 I: قالك واحد الطرف دلحم كيقطعوه ما كيرجعشي
He says that it is a piece of flesh that they remove, and it doesn't return

56 D: Y ya no tiene tiroides, entonces no puede aumentar el tamaño porque ya no tiene
And she no longer has a thyroid, so it cannot increase in size because she no longer has

57. I: نتنا حيدو لك تيرويديس، ويلا ماكاينشي ما يقدارشي يخلق،
هو كيخلق من التيرويديس
They have taken out your thyroid, and if there is none it can't be born, it is born of the thyroid

58 P: من العنق ديالي (????)قلو هادي ست شهور وانا هايدا
Tell him I take this way six months (????) of my neck

59 I: Ella dice que a veces me siento como mareada y mal y ella cree … y es lo que le digo que el tiroides no puede claro, es lo que le explico y ella no me hace caso
She says that sometimes I feel dizzy and sick, and she believes… and it is what I tell her that it can't be the thyroid …, right, it is what I explain to her, but she doesn't pay me attention

In this example we see that the husband is including information that neither the patient nor the doctor has given (55, 59). They are personal remarks based on information he has about the patient. The interpreter seems to act as the patient's advocate, counselling her and adding or omitting information. (For further references about the distinction between the advocacy and the impartial model, see Cambridge 2003: 57–59.) There are no examples of role changes of this kind in Type-3 consultations.

3.3 Changes in the interaction order

The general structure of doctor–patient interaction is usually that of an interview organized so as to include the following activities (see Heath 1992: 237; Borrell i Carrió 1999):

- Initial greetings
- Enunciation of problems
- Evaluation and discussion of the patient's condition
- Discussion and prescription of the treatment and/or of check-ups
- Farewells

Two other common characteristics studied by Díaz (1999) in oncological interviews and also considered in a previous study of monolingual medical encounters (Valero Garcés 2002) are:

- casual inserts or 'circumstantial conversation', made up of comments on topics or aspects of daily life not related to the medical consultation;
- bureaucratic negotiations, or comments by the doctor to help the patient solve difficulties related to the institution (comments on how to fill out forms, explanations on how to get a prescription or check-up, instructions on how to request an appointment with a specialist, etc.).

In the corpus under study, these features are more frequently used and rather longer in the case of Type-1 consultations, as was seen in Excerpt 1. They are not as frequent in Type-2 encounters, where the ad hoc interpreter has usually been in the country for some years and knows how the institutions work and is thus also familiar with the bureaucracy of healthcare institutions. However, there are examples where the general structure is changed, for example when talking about symptoms or treatment, as in Excerpt 3 (from C3):

Excerpt 3
72 D: El jarabe lo tiene que tomar si tiene ganas de vomitar
        She needs to take the syrup if she feels like vomiting
73 I: Solamente, ¿no?
        Only then, right?
74 D: Si con estas cápsulas se le quitan las ganas de vomitar no hace

75   I: *If she doesn't feel like vomiting while taking these pills, then she doesn't*

                                                                  No

       D (cont'd.): falta que tome el jarabe, pero ahora que siga tomándolo ¿eh?

       need to take the syrup, but for now she should keep taking it. Okay?

76   I: ¿Ahora sí?

       Now, yes?

77   D: Ahora sí. Si se le quitan las ganas de vomitar que lo deje

       Now, yes. If she doesn't feel like vomiting, then she can stop

78   I: فهمتي قالك هاد الخارابي شربو غير ملي يكون عندك غاناس دي بوميتار

                 دابا شربو   .ملي يحيدلك ما تبقاشي تشربو

       You know, he says to take this syrup only when you have to throw up, when

       you don't feel like it you can stop; take it now

The doctor explains three times (72, 74, 77) that the woman can stop taking the syrup "if she doesn't feel like vomiting", whereas the interpreter only relays this to the patient after the second repetition, and not without omitting some of the information.

There are no such examples of changes in the interaction order in Type-3 consultations. There, when the patient asks for information, it is usually related to the reason for the consultation. Furthermore, the interpreter may ask for clarification or repetition, as seen in Excerpt 4 (from C5):

Excerpt 4

90   D: Now, just one more comment about … um … because Chlamydia is a sexually transmitted disease … um … it is reported and … um … someone may be calling you. They may not. That … I'll just write something to the Department of Health stating that you have been treated, so you probably won't be contacted. However, um … because it is a sexually transmitted disease, we also want to offer to you HIV testing …

91   I: Hang on. I'm sorry.

92   D: That's right. Too much. Um … where do I want to start? Um … Do you want to tell her what you want to and then … or should I … um … okay, we'll back up. Um …

Another change in the general structure of the interview is associated with the use of extralinguistic resources by the doctor. In the treatment section of the two Type-1 consultations (C1, C2), strategies such as repetition, the use of notes, or drawings on a piece of paper generally accompany the doctor's explanations so as to ensure that the patient has understood.

In the case of triadic exchanges mediated by an ad hoc interpreter (Type 2), the same strategies are present — doctor's repetitions, reformulations, yes/no questions — making the consultation longer and harder to follow, as shown in Excerpt 5 (from C4):

Excerpt 5

95   D: ¿De cuándo son los análisis?
From when are the tests?

96   I: دشمن شهر؟
From what month?

97   P: قولو(؟؟؟؟)   قولو راه كاملين كتبو هو ملك واعطاوهم لك   شمن شهر؟
What month? From every month she has bring here, with you

98   I: De todos meses ella tienes traído aquí, contigo
From every month she has bring here, with you

99   D: Ya, pero los últimos ¿de cuándo son?
Okay, but the last ones. from when are they?

100   I: وقاش شبرتهم؟
The third month?

101   D: Del mes tres
The month three

102   P: شي، شي شهر هيداك
About a month ago

103   I: Un mes, un mes está en casa
One month, one month she is home

104   D: ¿Hace un mes sólo?
Only one month ago?

105   I: Sí
Yes

106   D: ¿Tiene análisis?
Does she have tests?

107   I: Sí
Yes

108   P: (????)

109   I: Si quiere, tráelo
If you want, bring it

110   D: Yo quiero verlos
I want to see them.

In the above example, D formulates his first question twice (95, 99), then asks for confirmation (104), and finally uses a direct statement (110) that sounds like an order to explain what he wants and thus finish this exchange. As for the interpreter, he answers the doctor's questions and generates new ones, without relaying them to the patient (except once, in turn 96). Finally the interpreter makes an offer (109) that could pragmatically be considered an order because of the linguistic form used, indicating a certain lack of knowledge of the contact language, in this case Spanish.

3.4 Changes in the contribution types

Some parts of interactions conducted in institutional settings are associated with specific discourse sequences, including series of routine activities performed by the respective participants (Drew & Heritage 1992; Drew & Sorjonen 1997; Heritage 1995, 1997). This means that, depending on the service provided by the institution or the moment of the interaction, specific linguistic forms are expected. Thus, in the medical evaluation section, the interaction is characterised by question–answer sequences, in which the question is a routine formula used by the supplier of services and the answer is provided by the patient. In this sense, the doctor usually tries to get information, and this function is generally performed with questions that can vary in form — direct or indirect — and may also involve the manipulation of intonation. At times the doctor may offer a list of options, but more often the patient will be told what to do, using the imperative, the immediate future, or the present. When the doctor speaks of bureaucratic negotiations s/he usually gives advice, and often uses conditional sentences or other linguistic structures associated with this function.

Concentrating on question–answer sequences in triadic exchanges (Type 2 and Type 3), the corpus analysis yields the quantitative findings summarised in Table 1.

Table 1. Questions by participants and interpreters' actions following the questions

	Total no. of questions	Doctor	Patient	Interpreter
C3	9	8	1	5 answered directly (56%) 2 translated (22%) 3 new questions
C4	28	25	3	12 answered directly (43%) 3 translated (11%) 4 new questions
C5	30	24	5	All translated, 1 new question
C6	31	28	3	All translated

Out of a total of 9 questions, the ad hoc interpreter in C3 answers 5 directly (56%) and translates only 2 (22%), while asking 3 new questions. Similarly, in C4, he answers 12 questions out of 25 (43%), translates only 2 (11%) and asks 4 new questions. In both Type-3 consultations, in contrast, the interpreter translates all questions, and in one instance asks for clarification.

Other changes that are common in Type-1 and Type-2 consultations are accommodation processes seen in the utterances of both doctors and ad hoc interpreters. In the case of the doctor, these include: short sentences; simplified language; more careful pronunciation; formulation of alternative questions (either ... or); formulation of yes/no (direct) questions; generic vocabulary and avoidance of technical terms; ungrammatical sentences, with omission of articles, prepositions and auxiliary verbs, or the use of infinitives instead of conjugated verb forms; frequent reformulation; and moves to take/recapture the initiative.

In our corpus these strategies are illustrated in Excerpts 6 (from C1) and 7 (from C3).

Excerpt 6

22 D: ¿Qué trabajas?
     What do you work?

23 P: Hoy descanso
     Today rest

24 D: Hoy descanso... ¿qué trabajas todos los días?
     Today rest... What do you work every day?

25 P: No, dos ó tres horas... siete por la mañana tres horas
     No, two or three hours ... seven in the morning three hours

26 D: ¿Vas a las siete y estás tres horas...?
     You go at seven and you are there for three hours ... ?

27 P: Yo ... por la mañana desde las siete hasta las tres
     Me ... in the morning from seven o'clock to three o'clock.

28 D: Vas a las siete hasta las tres... O sea trabajas de siete a tres
     You go from seven o'clock to three o'clock ... That is to say you work from seven to three

29 P: Sí, sí
     Yes, yes

30 D: O sea 7 a.m. a 3 p.m. ((writes this on a piece of paper and shows it to P)) ¿vale?
     So, 7 a.m. to 3 p.m.
     Okay?

31 P: Sí, sí
     Yes, yes

32 D: ¿Todos los días? ¿menos uno o dos libres a la semana?
     Every day? Except one or two days off a week?

33 P: Uno a la semana fiesta. Hoy descanso.
     One a week free. Today rest.

Thus, the doctor in Excerpt 6 uses simplified, colloquial language, even ungrammatical sentences (22), and reformulates the non-native-speaker patient's words (24, 30). His questions are direct, requiring simple answers (26, 32).

Examples of this kind are also found in Type-2 consultations. In Excerpt 7 (from C3), the doctor gives an explanation using three different forms (90):

Excerpt 7

88   D: Vale. ¿Usted tiene pastillas para no tener niños?
            Okay. You have pills for not having babies?

89   I: Sí, sí
           Yes, yes

90   D: Bueno, las pastillas disminuyen, hacen más pequeña la regla, menos sangre; ¿Lo entiende?
            Good, the pills lighten, make your period smaller, less blood. Do you understand?

91   I: Um
           Uh huh

92   D: Y esto está bien para el hierro. Está bien. Además no puede tener niños, que es lo que queremos
            And this is good for her iron. It's good. Besides she can't have babies, which is what we want

93   I: Vale
           Okay

94   I: Sí. ((to his wife))
           كيعملك الباستيات باش ميهبطولكش الدم بزاف وما يكونوش عندك الدراري
           Yes. ((to his wife)) He will give you pills so that there won't be much blood and don't catch
           ((to D)) ¿Pastillas menos sangre y no coge el el niños, ¿no? Vale
           ((to D)) Pills less blood and don't catch … babies, right? Okay.

The ad hoc interpreter, like the non-native-speaker patient in the monolingual interview, introduces questions, provides short answers, occasionally uses monosyllabic utterances, and sometimes does not even answer unless the doctor insists, or else, he provides more information than required and uses ungrammatical utterances with abundant repetition.

In Type-3 exchanges, the processes of accommodation by both the doctor and the patient are less evident; the doctor uses more technical words, and does not usually repeat or reformulate information. As for the interpreter, she still has some problems with language, and her translations are sometimes too literal and inaccurate. Excerpt 8 (from C5) illustrates some of these difficulties:

Excerpt 8

36   D: Well, I'm going to be giving you some medicine for you … to take.

37   I: Y le voy a dar medicamentos para que usted tome
           And I'm going to give you some medicine for you to take

38   D: And your partner will also need to be treated

39   I: Y su compañero va a necesitar tratamiento
           And your partner is also going to need treatment

40   P: ¿Por qué mi compañero?

> *Why my partner?*
> 41 I: And why my partner?
> 42 D: This is an infection that we know is passed sexually
> 43 I: Esta es una infección que es pasada sexualmente
>   *This is an infection that is passed sexually*

In the above example the doctor offers the patient clear information, using short sentences and avoiding specialised language. The interpreter translates literally, sometimes producing deviant utterances in Spanish (43).

3.5 Variation in lexical choice

Heritage (1997: 167) also states that the type of lexical choice made by participants in an institutional setting is indicative of the understanding and handling of the situation and of the speakers' command of the language (codes, styles, general or specific terms) as well as their awareness of the Other.

The use of appropriate vocabulary contributes to making communication more effective, but in the case of non-native-speaker patients and ad hoc interpreters who are not fluent in the language, this task is extremely difficult. The tendency is then to use generic terms, repetition, borrowings, invention of new words, code switching, or an inconsistent mix of registers. The rate of use of these resources is generally related to an asymmetry of knowledge between the patient and the doctor, on the one hand, and to problems derived from an incomplete knowledge of the language, on the other. Some examples found are: '*examen de oreja y ojo*' ('ear and eye examinations') instead of '*examen de vista y oído*' ('hearing and eyesight examinations'), or 'cuando abrimos la television`' ('when we open the television') instead of '*cuando ponemos la television*' ('when we turn on the TV'), or the use of very colloquial expressions, as in '*yo tengo de cuidar una vieja*' ('I have to watch that old lady'), using highly colloquial Spanish to refer to an elderly woman, instead of '*tengo que cuidar de una anciana*' ('I have to take care of an elderly woman').

In Type-3 consultations, there were no problems of this kind, although specialised terms and expressions also proved difficult for the interpreter, as can be seen in Excerpt 9 (from C5):

Excerpt 9
30 D: The discharge and also the pain ... the bleeding with intercourse
31 I: *El flujo y también el sangramiento cuando tiene relaciones*
          The discharge and also the bleeding when you have relations
32 D: *And the pain with intercourse you're having*
          Y el dolor cuando tiene relaciones sexuales
33 I: *Y el dolor cuando tiene relaciones también.*

In this exchange, we find words such as 'discharge', 'bleeding', and 'intercourse', terms which can be considered specialized if the context in which they were used is taken into account. The translation strategies used are a literal translation for 'discharge' and 'bleeding', with different results. The translation 'flujo' is acceptable, while *sangramiento* does not exist in Spanish, and the translation for 'intercourse' (*relaciones*) is incomplete since it does not specify what kind of relations are meant.

Generally speaking, we could say that, in all three types of encounters, the doctor sometimes tries to adapt his/her speech to the patients' command of the language by replacing technical terms with descriptive words, synonyms, repetitions, direct forms, and even ungrammatical sentences; that is, the doctor tries to offset or to reduce the communicative distance by adapting the grammar and vocabulary to both the patient's and the interpreter's knowledge of the language.

4. Quantitative comparison

Some similarities and differences can be distinguished and quantified by comparing the pattern and content of monolingual interviews (Type 1 — C1, C2) to the two interpreted interview types (Type 2 — C3, C4; Type 3 — C5, C6). Table 2 provides information about the total number of speaker turns in each recorded conversation as well as the rate of participation of each participant.

Table 2. Speaker turns in C1–C6

	C1	C2	C3	C4	C5	C6
Doctor	98	70	31	41	71	78
	(55%)	(54%)	(39%)	(37%)	(37%)	(31%)
Patient	79	60	13	21	28	73
	(45%)	(46%)	(16%)	(19%)	(14%)	(29%)
Ad hoc Interpreter			36	48		
			(45%)	(44%)		
Trained Interpreter					94	99
					(49%)	(40%)
Total	177	130	80	110	193	250
	(100%)	(100%)	(100%)	(100%)	(100%)	(100%)

As seen in Table 2, the number of turns in the monolingual interviews shows a similar distribution between doctor and patient, with the former producing 8%–10% more turns. In Type-2 encounters, the largest share of turns is recorded for the ad hoc interpreter, who is responsible for a higher percentage of turns (44%–

45%) than the trained interpreter in C6 (40%). In C5, nearly 50% of the turns are produced by the interpreter, which is what one would expect if the interpreter rendered both the doctor's and the patient's utterances in the other language.

Obviously, the principal difference between the monolingual and the interpreted interviews is the amount of 'direct interaction' between doctor and patient. In the monolingual interviews, doctor and patient use the same language and therefore have the potential to understand one another. However, since the patient has only a limited command of the language and insufficient knowledge about administrative procedures, the monolingual, dyadic encounters show processes of accommodation as well as changes in interaction patterns and in the distribution of time and roles.

In the case of the triadic interviews, the only way to establish verbal interaction between doctor and patient is through the bilingual husband acting as ad hoc interpreter (C3, C4) and through the hospital interpreter (C5, C6). Thus, only those utterances by the bilingual agent that are interpretations of another's speech constitute "direct interaction" between the doctor and the patient in these interviews. In Type-2 encounters, however, the ad hoc interpreter not only translates, but also adds or omits information or gives advice, while in Type 3, the interpreter mainly reproduces what the doctor and patient say in the other language. This was seen in the quantitative analysis of questions and their fate in the bilingual mediated encounters (see Table 1). In Type-2 consultations, only 5 of the 37 questions (14%) were translated, while in Type 3, all the questions asked by the doctor were interpreted directly to the patient.

5. Conclusion

The comparative analysis of dyadic and triadic doctor–patient consultations presented in this paper has yielded a number of relevant findings. In the monolingual mode (Type 1), while there is direct one-to-one communication between health-care professional and patient, the patient's limited language proficiency and lack of institutional knowledge result in changes in the assignment of participant roles, in the interaction order and in the contribution types. Similar phenomena can be observed in Type 2 encounters: The ad hoc interpreter's linguistic competence is not very high, although he has better knowledge of how the institution works and some other interactional resources, which tend to reduce the occurrence of bureaucratic explanations or casual inserts. Nevertheless, the rate of direct one-to-one communication is quite low, as the husband-interpreter moves freely between the roles of interpreter, patient advocate and husband, frequently taking over the doctor's role of questioning and counselling the patient or providing information about the patient directly to the doctor. Whenever the ad hoc interpreter speaks directly to either the doctor or the patient, no interpretation is available to the other party, and replies are often not translated.

Finally, in Type-3 consultations, mediated by a trained hospital interpreter, the bilingual third party was found to be quite skilled in interpreting and to maintain a narrowly defined interpreter role. However, there was evidence of some problems with terminology and with memory for longer stretches of discourse.

Comparison between the three types of encounters also indicates that Type 1 and Type 2 share some features related to the use of certain communication strategies (frequent questions, repetitions, reformulations, etc.) and that these affect the general structure of the interview and the participants' roles. In the case of Type 2, the ad hoc interpreter acts more as an advocate and husband than solely as an interpreter. While his failure to relay utterances by the doctor and the patient to the other participant may save time, it constitutes a considerable communicative risk: the doctor feels that the husband knows his wife's (i.e. the patient's) problem but he cannot be sure about the husband's skill and ability to interpret accurately and hence often uses similar resources as in the monolingual interview (Type 1).

The interpreter in the two Type-3 encounters maintains an impartial role and uses specific strategies such as direct rendition of questions or asking for reformulation when she has difficulties (e.g. with terminology or long utterances). Thus, whereas the ad hoc interpreter fails to translate or avoids technical terms (e.g. using "back" when the doctor says "spine"), the hospital interpreter asks the doctor for clarification. The trained interpreter also uses the first person, whereas in consultations involving an ad hoc interpreter the three participants frequently use the third person ('tell her', 'ask her', 'she says').

In conclusion, this study illustrates some differences and similarities between three different types of interaction between doctors and immigrant patients with some or practically no command of the official language: monolingual vs. bilingual, mediated either by an ad hoc interpreter or by a trained hospital interpreter. Though most of the study is descriptive, it also serves as a reminder of the importance of using professional interpreters in medical consultations. Furthermore, the use of examples taken from this corpus can be valuable for educational purposes, both in the training of future healthcare interpreters and in initiatives to help doctors work effectively with interpreters.

Notes

1. The research carried out for the writing of this paper is part of two projects, one funded by the University of Alcalá (Ref. UAH OI 2004/010) and focused on the quality of communication between healthcare staff and foreign patients at one of the biggest hospitals in Madrid, and the other (still in progress) funded by the Spanish Ministry of Education (Ref. HUM2004-03774-C02-02-FILO) (2004–2007) and centred on the quality of communication between healthcare staff and foreign patients and on the development of proposals for training. I also want to thank Franz Pöchhacker, Brook Townsley and two anonymous reviewers for their helpful comments.

2. Since the creation of FITISPos (*Formación e Investigación en Traducción e Interpretación en los Servicios Públicos* / Training and Research in Public Service Translation and Interpreting) in 1998, the corpus has been extended, thanks to several research projects funded by public or private institutions.

3. The numbers in the examples indicate the turn in the conversation. The translation offered is a literal one, reflecting as much as possible the often nonstandard use of Spanish in the original. The transcription code, which for the sake of readability has been reduced to a minimum, is as follows:

(????)	unintelligible
?	interrogative rising intonation
…	pause
((…))	extralinguistic comment
}	overlapping

References

Borrell i Carrió, F. (1999). *Manual de entrevista clínica*. Barcelona: Doyma.

Cambridge, J. (2003). Unas ideas sobre la interpretación en los centros de salud. In C. Valero Garcés (Ed.), *Traducción e interpretación en los servicios públicos. Contextualización, actualidad y futuro*. Granada: Comares, 51–70.

Davidson, B. (2002). A model for the construction of conversational common ground in interpreted discourse. *Journal of Pragmatics* 34, 1273–1300.

Díaz, F. (1999). Asimetría profesional en la consulta de oncología: algunas constricciones conversacionales de la clínica. *Discurso y Sociedad* 1 (4), 35–68.

Drew, P. & Heritage, J. (Eds.) (1992). *Talk at work*. Cambridge: Cambridge University Press.

Drew, P. & Sorjonen, M. L. (1997). Institutional dialogue. In T. A. van Dijk (Ed.), *Discourse as Social Interaction*. London: Sage, 91–118.

Heath, C. (1992). The delivery and reception of diagnosis in the general-practice consultation. In P. Drew & J. Heritage (Eds.), *Talk at work*, Cambridge: Cambridge University Press, 235–267.

Heritage, J. (1995). Conversation analysis: Methodological aspects. In U. M. Quasthoff (Ed.), *Aspects of oral communication*. Berlin: de Gruyter, 391–418.

Heritage, J. (1997). Conversation analysis and institutional talk. In D. Silverman (Ed.), *Qualitative Research: Theory, Method and Practice*. London: Sage, 161–182.

Mason, I. (Ed.) (2001). *Triadic exchanges. Studies in dialogue interpreting*. Manchester: St. Jerome.

Meyer, B. (2001). How untrained interpreters handle medical terms. In I. Mason (Ed.), *Triadic exchanges. Studies in dialogue interpreting*. Manchester: St Jerome, 87–106.

Meyer, B., Apfelbaum, B., Pöchhacker, F. & Bischoff, A. (2003). Analysing interpreted doctor–patient communication from the perspectives of linguistics, interpreting studies and health sciences. In L. Brunette, G. Bastin, I. Hemlin & H. Clarke (Eds.), *The critical link* 3. Amsterdam/Philadelphia: John Benjamins, 66–79.

Valero Garcés, C. (2001). Estudio para determinar el tipo y calidad de la comunicación lingüística con la población extranjera en los Centros de Salud." *OFRIM, Suplementos* 9 (diciembre 2001), 117–132.

Valero Garcés, C. (2002). Interaction and conversational constrictions in the relationships between suppliers of services and immigrant users. *Pragmatics* 12 (4), 469–496.

Valero Garcés, C. (2003). Talk, work, and institutional order: Processes of accommodation in doctor/immigrant patient interaction. In I. Palacios Martínez et al. (Eds.), *Fifty years of English Studies in Spain (1952–2002). A commemorative*. Santiago de Compostela: Universidad de Santiago de Compostela, Vol. I, 663–670.

Wadensjö, C. (1992). *Interpreting as interaction. On dialogue interpreting in immigration hearings and medical encounters*. Linköping: Linköping University.

Exploring untrained interpreters' use of direct versus indirect speech

Friedel Dubslaff and Bodil Martinsen
Aarhus School of Business

This study examines the interrelations between the use of direct vs. indirect speech by primary participants and by dialogue interpreters by focusing on pronoun shifts and their interactional functions. The data consist of four simulated interpreter-mediated medical interviews based on the same scripted role play. The subjects were untrained Arabic interpreters working for a Danish agency. Two of the four interpreters favoured the direct style of interpreting. The other two favoured the indirect style. The findings show that all four interpreters tended to identify with the patient by personalizing the indefinite pronoun *one* when relaying from doctor to patient. All other pronoun shifts occurred in connection with interactional problems caused almost exclusively by the interpreters' lack of knowledge about medical terminology — even though the terms used were in fact non-specialized ones. The study also indicates that primary parties' shifts from direct to indirect address are closely related either to the form or to the content of the interpreter's prior utterance. Finally, it emerges that repeated one-language talk, triggered by the interpreter's problems with medical terminology, can override the quasi-directness of communication between primary participants, which is connected with interpreting in the first person.

Introduction

Since 1999, the authors of the present paper have been involved in testing untrained interpreters with migrant languages at the Aarhus School of Business. During the oral test, which includes an interview about the role of the interpreter and interpreting ethics, interpreters sometimes stated which style they favoured: the first-person style or the third-person style. However, in the subsequent role play, they did not always adhere to their avowed preference. Consequently, the authors of the present study wondered what made the interpreters deviate from the style they claimed to use, and decided to explore their use of direct vs. indirect speech.

There is general agreement in the literature that interpreters should use the speaker's first person (direct speech) when rendering the utterances of primary participants in face-to-face encounters. Handbooks and guidelines explaining professional practice to beginners, untrained practitioners and/or professional clients provide ample evidence of this (e.g. Adams et al. 1995; Gentile et al. 1996; Galal & Galal 1999; Phelan 2001; Baaring 2001; Domstolsstyrelsen 2003), as do accounts of interpreting in publications directed at scholars within Translation Studies (e.g. Wadensjö 1998a). Thus, the first person is regarded as the norm followed by professional interpreters (Harris 1990; Wadensjö 1998b; Pöchhacker 2004; Hale 2004) and exceptions to this norm are explicitly mentioned as such (Shlesinger 1991: 152; Gentile et al. 1996: 25–26, 88; Meyer 2002: 53).

In contrast, so-called natural interpreters or lay interpreters tend to use the third person (indirect speech) in community interpreting (Shackman 1984; Knapp & Knapp-Potthoff 1985). Third-person style is thus regarded as the norm in this context (Harris 1990; Pöchhacker 2004). Exceptions are found in e.g. Shackman (1984), who maintains that direct vs. indirect style is partly a matter of personal preference.

The rationale behind the direct mode of interpreting

According to the literature, the most obvious advantage of the first-person style is that it enhances the directness of communication between the primary participants (e.g. Baaring 2001; Razban 2003; Hale 2004), or, more precisely, that it helps create and maintain "the illusion of a direct exchange between the monolingual parties" (Wadensjö 1997: 49).

Other advantages are the enhancement of accuracy (Hale 2004), clarity (Galal & Galal 1999; Driesen 2002), brevity (Lings 1988; Baaring 2001), impartiality (Niska 1999; Baaring 2001), mutual understanding between primary interlocutors (Galal & Galal 1999), a common focus of interaction (Wadensjö 1997) and a non-dominating and less-manipulating behaviour (Lings 1988).

There is no doubt then that the direct mode of interpreting is generally regarded as superior to the indirect.

The aim of the study

As mentioned above, the present study focuses on untrained practitioners' use of direct vs. indirect speech. More specifically, the aim is to explore (1) the interactional functions of interpreters' choice of particular pronouns;[1] (2) the interrelation between interpreters' and the primary participants' choice of pronouns; and (3) factors that may affect the superiority of the first-person style.

The issue of interpreters' use of direct vs. indirect speech is by no means new (Mason 1999: 152), but few studies have focused solely on this aspect (e.g. Bot 2003 and this volume).

Our study will centre on pronoun shifts as illustrations of how participants change their *footing* (Goffman 1981). Within Goffman's participation framework, *footing* is "the alignment we and others present adopt, as expressed in the way we manage the production or reception of an utterance" (1981: 128). In our analysis of the data we will draw upon Wadensjö's (1998b) expanded model of this framework, which complements Goffman's notion of a production format (animator, author, principal) with a corresponding notion of a reception format (reporter, recapitulator, responder).

When discussing examples from the data, we shall also draw upon Wadensjö's (1998b: 107–108) taxonomy of interpreter utterances. Wadensjö uses the following definitions — to mention only the categories applied in the present study:

-   In a '*close rendition*' "the propositional content found explicitly expressed in the 'rendition' must be equally found in the preceding 'original', and the style of the two utterances should be approximately the same [in principle]";
-   An '*expanded rendition*' "includes more explicitly expressed information than the preceding 'original' utterance";
-   A '*reduced rendition*' "includes less explicitly expressed information than the preceding 'original' utterance";
-   A '*substituted rendition*' "consists of a combination of an 'expanded' and a 'reduced' one";
-   A '*summarized rendition*' "is a text that corresponds to two or more prior 'originals.'" The originals may be provided by the same or by different individuals and sometimes "an interpreter's utterance and an 'original' can together provide the information summarized in a succeeding 'rendition.'"
-   A '*non-rendition*' "is a 'text' which is analysable as an interpreter's initiative or response which does not correspond (as translation) to a prior 'original' utterance".

Data collection

Test material

The data analysed in this study comprises four simulated doctor-patient interviews. These data, originally collected during a test of interpreting skills and not for the purpose of the present or any other study, were found to present a number of advantages, deriving from the fact that the same scripted interview was conducted with the same primary parties under roughly the same conditions, but with different interpreters — thus allowing for inter-individual comparison. This is why it was decided to use them for the present purpose.

The simulated interviews did, however, contain one authentic feature: the "doctor" did not understand Arabic and she was thus in the same position as the majority of professional Danish healthcare providers who work with interpreters.

The script was constructed to test the basic interpreting skills of untrained practitioners employed on a freelance basis by the Danish Refugee Council's (DRC) interpreting service operating in the Western part of Denmark. As there are no proper interpreter training options outside the capital of Copenhagen, interpreting agencies in other parts of the country have no way of evaluating the skills of their interpreters. That is why the DRC initiated and paid for the testing of both their staff and freelance interpreters. An important part of the test was dedicated to simulated medical interviews such as the ones analysed here. The medical setting was chosen because the DRC interpreters work mainly within medical as well as social service settings.

When constructing the script for the interview, the testers chose (a) a common setting, i.e. an interview in a general practitioner's consultation; (b) a common topic, i.e. hypertension; and (c) common terms, i.e. Danish terms or "semi-professional expressions" (Meyer 2001) rather than highly specialized medical terminology. The testers thus assumed that the interpreter's task in this interview would be fairly simple — an assumption that turned out to be incorrect, as will be demonstrated below.

As a source of inspiration for the construction of the script, the researchers used the description of hypertension by two medical doctors on the Danish website NetDoktor (Gill & Kristensen, no year). The script was submitted to a general practitioner for evaluation to ensure that it did not contain errors and that it was a reasonable reflection of real-life medical consultations. Its structure was in keeping with the following standard stages of medical interviews (applied e.g. by Metzger 1999: 59):

1. Opening
2. Medical history
3. Examination
4. Diagnosis
5. Consultation
6. Medical advice.

These stages will be referred to again in the discussion of examples from the recorded data.

Frames

The actual testing was carried out in a meeting room at the Aarhus School of Business by one of the authors of this paper and by a certified community interpreter of Arabic.[2] Six interpreters participated in the oral test on the day in question. Before the test, the interpreters were asked whether they would be willing to support a research project by consenting to an audio-recording of their performance in the role play. The purpose of the study was also presented to them, but in very general terms. All six interpreters consented.

The interpreted conversations to be analysed are a complex type of encounter. As illustrated by Figure 1 (an adaptation of Metzger 1999), there are many different frames or perspectives, all of which have some bearing on the data.

The testers were also the primary participants in the role play: one of the authors of this paper played the role of the doctor, and the Arabic community interpreter played the patient. Presumably, this exam-like situation was intensified by the co-presence of the employer from the DRC agency, though he was there only as an observer. He also used the test as an opportunity to acquaint himself with the freelance interpreters whom he had never actually met. Thus, his status, in Goffman's terms (1981: 135) can be described as "neither ratified participation nor bystanding, but a peculiar condition between." A similar participation status could be ascribed to the second author of this paper, who was present taking notes during the testing of only two interpreters in the present study.

In discussing the naturalness of her recorded (authentic) data, Wadensjö (1998b: 95) points out that the presence of a researcher may sometimes make professional interpreters feel that they are in a test situation, which again may make them try "to do what they understand to be best." There is reason to believe that the test frame in combination with the research frame had a similar effect on the interpreters in this study. Example 1 below thus may illustrate the dominance of the test frame. (For an explanation of the transcription conventions used in the

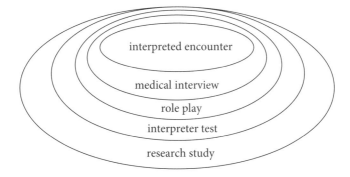

Figure 1. Frames (after Metzger 1999: 57 and 69)

extracts, see *Transcriptions and translations* at the end of the section on the *Categorization of data.*)

At this point in the interview, the doctor (D) has formulated her diagnosis that the patient (P) is suffering from moderately elevated blood pressure. P now wants to know whether he should take medication for his condition, and D explains that this is not necessarily the case.

Example 1
D   21b Der er mange ting man **selv** kan gøre og hvis det hjælper så er der ingen grund til at tage medicin.
There are many things one can do oneself and if that helps then there is no reason to take medicine.
I(B) →   Nej, men hvad skal han gøre så?
No, but what has he got to do then?
D   Ja det (.) det kan vi snakke om bagefter.
Well that (.) we can talk about that later.

The interpreter I(B) does not translate D's answer but responds directly by posing a new question on behalf of P. This seems to indicate I(B)'s strong involvement in the interaction and possibly also his wish to perform well in the test by being "ahead" of the primary participants' talk. (See Example 4 for a more elaborate discussion of this exchange).

Methodology

In the script, the doctor and the patient never use the third person form of address (*he/she*) but — following Wadensjö's categorization (1997: 48) — do occasionally use other forms of indirect address, such as the indefinite pronoun *man* (*one*), as in Example 1.

The script comprises 44 turns.[3] The patient, with 20 turns, uses a direct form in addressing the doctor — corresponding to the use of *you*, second person singular — in two successive turns, and no address in the other turns. The doctor, with 24 turns, uses direct address in 15 turns and the simultaneously direct and indirect address, i.e. the institutional *vi* (*we*) including the speaker (Wadensjö 1997), in one turn. In four of the remaining turns, she uses no address, and in another four turns, she uses the indefinite *man* (*one).*

Evidently, based on the above, the interpreters' use of the third-person indirect *he/she*-form during the role play was generally not influenced by the utterances of the primary participants. Nor was it affected by the official policy of the DRC agency, which distributes an informational brochure to new freelance interpreters, explaining the advantages of the direct style and recommends its use (Dansk Flygtningehjælp 2001: 4).

Since the DRC agency merely recommends the direct style but does not prescribe it, interpreters are free to choose. Consequently, the interpreters' shifts from direct to indirect style and vice versa in the present study were explored by identifying instances where they deviated from their preferred style.

As for the primary participants, they were expected to play their roles according to the script that had been written out in both Danish and Arabic. Some improvisation was allowed in order to ensure the necessary flexibility within the role play and the test frame, but the primary participants were expected to return to the script as soon as possible and to follow the instructed form of address throughout. Their deviations from the style of address used in the script will also be explored below.

Criteria for the selection of subjects

For practical reasons, the first selection criterion was the foreign language. Arabic was chosen because it was possible to recruit an independent qualified native speaker of Arabic to help with the transcriptions and the translations of the turns. The second criterion — the same tester and co-tester in the role play — has already been mentioned. The third criterion was an equal number of (almost) consistent users of the direct and the indirect styles, respectively. For the sake of inter-group comparison, at least four subjects were needed, two using the direct style of interpreting and two using the indirect. The criterion *untrained* was given beforehand, because the agency would not test graduates of academic interpreting programmes.

Table 1 provides some basic information about the four subjects. For the sake of anonymity, few details are given about their personal background.

Table 1. Subjects

Subject	Preferred style	Interpreter experience	Interpreter training	Educational background
A male age 24	direct	some	none	student at college of education in Denmark (Danish, social studies)
C female age 29	direct	very little	undergraduate T&I course in the Middle East (no certificate)	lower secondary school in Denmark, GCSE in the Middle East
B male age ca. 30	indirect	some	none	agricultural school in Denmark; mother-tongue: Kurdish
D male age 36	indirect	some	none	electrical engineer (Eastern Europe)

The fact that one of the subjects, I(C), had participated briefly in a T&I course was not considered a disqualifying factor for the purpose of the present study. Like the other subjects, I(C) does not hold a degree in interpreting and/or translation, or a certificate in community interpreting. Besides, her T&I course was in English and Arabic, which puts her on an equal footing with the other subjects with respect to Danish. Nevertheless, her T&I course had most probably acquainted I(C) with some basic interpreting techniques, such as the use of direct style.[4]

It must be assumed that their educational background has provided I(C) as well as I(A) with a certain number of language skills, as well as with language awareness, which may have contributed to their performance as community interpreters. I(B) and I(D) apparently had only limited language training. Moreover, I(B) was not a native speaker of Arabic, which may be regarded as a disadvantage in an Arabic test.

Categorization of data

Tables 2 and 3 provide an overview of the number and types of pronoun shifts found in each of the four interviews.

Table 2. Number and types of interpreters' pronoun shifts

1 Inter- preter	2 1st→3rd	3 3rd→1st	4 1st or 3rd →1st self	5 (D3 rd)→2nd	6 (D3rd)→1st pl.
A *	3	–	0	3	0
C *	2	–	4	1	0
B **	–	2	1	1	0
D **	–	0	0	3	1

Legend: * = direct style, ** = indirect style; D3rd: doctor's impersonal pronoun

Table 3. Number and types of primary participants' pronoun shifts

Inter- preter	doctor's shift 2nd → 3rd	patient's shift 2nd → 3rd
A *	1	1
C *	2	1
B **	12	0
D **	2	1

Table 2 lists the interpreters' pronoun shifts. The first column shows in which interview the pronoun shifts occur and indicates the preferred style of the interpreter involved. Column 2 lists the direct-style interpreters' shifts from the first person to the third, while column 3 lists the indirect-style interpreters' shifts from the third person to the first. Column 4 lists another kind of interpreter shift, namely from the third person or from *I* meaning *other* to *I* meaning *self*.

The shifts in columns 5 and 6 are different from those in columns 2, 3 and 4, because they do not list deviations from an interpreter's own preferred style, but rather his/her rendering of the pronouns used by a primary participant, in this case the doctor — indicated as D3rd in brackets. Generally, these were shifts from the indefinite *man* (literally *one*) to the second person singular (column 5) or, in one instance, to the institutional first person plural (column 6).

Table 3 lists shifts from direct to indirect address in the utterances of the primary participants.

Interestingly, a kind of switch that did not occur in the data is from the conventional address, the Danish second person singular *du*, generally used in encounters in Denmark, to the polite address in Arabic (the second person plural), which would have been appropriate in the setting.[5] A possible explanation might be a lack of awareness, at least on the part of the three subjects who had never received any interpreter training.

Transcriptions and translations

The transcription conventions adopted for the present study follow the conventions in *The Translator* 5(2), 1999. Below, however, we have listed only the ones that do not appear to be self-evident from the examples discussed in the next section.

Thus, / marks an abandoned utterance, (xxx) an inaudible sequence, … indicates open-ended intonation, **boldface** indicates emphasis, (.) marks a short pause, (2) a two-second pause, and e:r a lengthened vowel sound (in a filled pause). For technical reasons, it was necessary to use underlined passages (instead of square brackets) to indicate overlapping talk.

As regards the English translations, all utterances, including medical terms, have been rendered literally — i.e. non-idiomatically — when this was considered necessary in order to make explicit what caused interlocutors' production and/or comprehension problems.

Discussion

The discussion of pronoun shifts will focus on the interpreters' change of footing, but will also include examples of the primary participants' change of footing.

Direct-style interpreters' change of footing

I(A) uses the first-person style almost consistently throughout the interview. In two of the three exceptions shown in Table 2, the data do not reveal any specific interactional function of the shift to the third person, whereas the exchange in Example 2 below illustrates a pronoun shift which seems to have a distancing function.

At this point in the interview, D informs P about the risks of high blood pressure, including cardiovascular diseases.

Example 2

D21e   Men der er en forøget risiko for hjerte-kar-sygdomme, og derfor skal man gøre noget ved det.
But there is an increased risk of heart and [blood] vessel diseases and therefore one has to do something about it.

Ia.   أ لكن أأ في الحقيقة أ هناك أ أرتفاع أ في نسبة خطر أن يصيبك مرض   قلبي، مرض في القلب
Er but e:r in reality there is er a higher percentage of a risk that you get a heart disease, a disease in the heart.

P   في القلب ... أ وين في القلب؟ أين؟
In the heart... er where in the heart? Where?

Ia.   أأ
e:r

P   أين في القلب؟ في أي جزء في القلب؟
Where in the heart? In which part in the heart?

I(A) →   Han spørger hvorhenne det er i hjertet øh at (.) at (1) at der kan ske noget.
He asks where it is in the heart er that (.) that (1) that something can happen.

The risk of cardiovascular diseases is rendered by I(A) as a risk of getting a "heart disease". Undoubtedly, the co-tester/patient notices that I(A) has provided a reduced rendition by omitting *vascular* diseases ("*kar*-sygdomme") and reacts to this. Moreover, the risk is emphasized by I(A)'s repetition ("a disease in the heart") and by his substitution of D's indefinite pronoun *one* for the personal *you* ("a risk that *you* get a heart disease") — for more about this type of rendition see Examples 4 and 5 below. In addition, I(A) omits the second part of D's utterance, namely that patients can do something to lessen the risk. As a result, P becomes quite upset and reacts by asking for clarification twice, uttering his questions at an accelerated pace and with a higher pitch, and without relinquishing the turn to I(A).

Presumably, I(A) did not know the term *kar* in "hjerte-kar-sygdomme" and therefore omitted it. His trouble rendering this expression may have caused his omission of the second part of D's utterance as well. If he is unaware of his omissions he may prefer a summarized rendition just because he feels uncomfortable providing a close rendition of P's emotional utterances which so clearly display distress in form and content. However, if he is aware of his omissions, he may opt not to transmit the emotions of P's utterances, knowing that he himself has actually caused them. He may also feel that omissions in a test situation are bound to cause him some anxiety. In any case, I(A) seemingly does not want to assume responsibility for P's utterances, and therefore chooses to summarize them indirectly, using the third person.

The other direct-style interpreter, I(C), shifts to the third person on two occasions, also resorting to summarized renditions. One of these is illustrated as Example 3 below. This incident is even more complex than I(A)'s shift above, because I(C) changes her footing three times within the summarizing turn. This is a striking illustration of Goffman's (1981: 128) statement whereby "Participants over the course of their speaking constantly change their footing."

Prior to the exchange in Example 3, D asks P "Are your parents still alive?" This question is one of a series of questions, the purpose of which is to establish P's medical history. The exchange starts with P's answer.

Example 3

P 17   فقط والدي (1) والدتي توفت من سنوات **عديدة** (2) حيث أصيبت
بإنسداد شريان (×××) وهذا مفتوح على (×××)

*Only my father (1) my mother died **many** years ago (2) as she got a blocked artery (xxx) and that er ends in (xxx)*

Ic.   والشريان التاجي ده وين (×××) ؟

And the coronary artery where is (xxx)?

P   في الألب

In the heart.

Ic.   في الألب؟

In the heart?

Ic.   أأأ والدك توفى (1) وإلا والدتك؟

E::r your father died (1) or your mother?

P   والدتي

My mother.

I(C) →   **والدتك ؟**

*[Your] **mother?***

> Ø:h min mor hun er **død** for mange år siden og hun døde på grund af (.)
> / han fortæller at (.) / jeg ved ikke hvad sygdommen er, men det er en åre
> der er blevet storknet til hjertet. Det var det jeg forstod af det.
> *E:r my mother she is **dead** many years ago and she died because of (.)/ he*
> *says that(.) / I don't know what the disease is but it is an artery which has*
> *got clotted to the heart. That is what I understood of it.*

D → Det var hans **mor**. Hvad med faderen?
*That was his **mother**. What about his father?*

Part of P's answer was inaudible, but I(C)'s request for clarification indicates that
he mentioned a term corresponding to *coronary artery*. Next, I(C) asks P to repeat
a piece of information, indicating that she either did not hear it, or had forgotten it.
Moreover, following each of P's answers, I(C) utters an echoic question — possibly
to gain more time for comprehension.

I(C) begins her rendition of P's answer in the first person ("my mother she is
dead"), but then she shifts to the third person ("He says that"). Her shift thus has a
distancing effect, similar to the one caused by I(A)'s shift in Example 2. I(C) then
shifts a third time, to the first person *I,* meaning herself, expressing her doubts
about her own rendering of what had caused the death of P's mother. She repeats
this doubt once more before finishing the turn.

Example 3 is interesting as regards the distribution of responsibility. As
Wadensjö (1993: 103) puts it, the dialogue interpreter "has, by definition, a certain
pregiven responsibility for the primary parties' attaining of shared knowledge."
I(C) is seemingly sensitive to this. She starts by disclaiming responsibility for P's
utterance, by means of the shift to the third person. However, she then shifts to the
first person *I,* meaning *self,* thus indicating that she is willing to take on at least
part of the responsibility herself. Her intensive use of hedges may be intended to
"compensate" for her "lack of knowledge about medical terminology" (Bührig &
Meyer 2004: 8). In contrast, her meta-talk about the meaning of P's utterance may
also be intended to convey the message that she blames the patient for not having
expressed himself in a comprehensible manner.

At the same time, this meta-talk demonstrates a change of the interpreter's
participation status. By referring explicitly and repeatedly to her own perception of P's utterances, I(C) becomes a primary participant on equal terms with D
— which has an impact on D's way of responding in the subsequent turn. Instead
of resuming the direct address of P in her question concerning P's father, D treats
I(C) as a primary interlocutor and thus as the ultimate addressee of her question
(see also Example 6 below).

To sum up, the interpreters' pronoun shifts in Examples 2 and 3 occurred in
summarized renditions of prior one-language talk. When summarizing these exchanges, the interpreters had to combine two conflicting perspectives: their own

and that of one of the primary participants. Thus, it seems that the main function of their shifts to the third person in the two examples was to disclaim responsibility for interactional problems.

Indirect-style interpreters' change of footing

Example 4 illustrates yet another summarized rendition, but there are no conflicting perspectives to be combined or rather, I(B), who is an almost consistent indirect-style interpreter,[6] is apparently not aware of a potential conflict, and the pronoun shift in question has a different function.

The prior talk between I(B) and D has already been cited as Example 1. At this point at the beginning of the consultation stage, P wants to know if he has to take medicine for his elevated blood pressure. D's first utterance in Example 4 is one of a series of utterances explaining this medical condition in general terms as well as the standard treatment options. As she speaks in general terms, D uses the indefinite *man* (*one*) and other impersonal linguistic devices rather than the direct-style address.

> **Example 4**
>
> D 21b   Der er mange ting man **selv** kan gøre og hvis det hjælper så er der ingen grund til at tage medicin.
> *There are many things one can do oneself and if that helps then there is no reason to take medicine.*
>
> Ib.   Nej, men hvad skal han gøre så?
> *No, but what has he got to do then?*
>
> D   Ja det (.) det kan vi snakke om bagefter.
> *Well that (.) we can talk about that later.*
>
> I(B) →   في بعض الأشياء الأخرى أ أ أنت تقدر تستعملها/ بعدين نحكي عنها
> *There are some other things e:r you can use yourself these / we will talk about them later.*

In Example 4, I(B) first takes on the role of responder instead of just translating D's utterance. Clearly, his question on behalf of P is disqualifying D's just provided utterance as a good enough reply to P's question. Possibly, D's use of the indirect form of address is what makes I(B) perceive himself as the ultimate addressee.

However, D does not let I(B) alter her agenda and refuses to answer his question. I(B) then provides a summarized rendition. Furthermore, instead of providing a close translation of D's indefinite *one*, which would have been possible as there are several common options for this in Arabic, I(B) addresses P directly and explicitly by using the Arabic pronoun *ante* corresponding to *you*, second person singular (cf. note 1). He is seemingly not aware of the communicative purpose underlying D's use of *one*, which is — as Bührig & Meyer (2004: 8) suggest in the context of briefings for informed consent — to underline "the professional and well-established character" of the treatment and thereby "to ensure the patient's cooperation and to establish a relationship of trust."

As can be seen from column 5 in Table 2, this type of "personalizing" of an utterance (Tebble 1999: 191) is used by all four interpreters. We have already seen one example in the exchange with I(A), who prefers the direct style (Example 2). However, it is interesting to note that the two indirect-style interpreters also choose direct address in their renditions of the indefinite *one*.

The preference for the direct address may reflect the interpreters' tendency to identify with the speaker of their mother tongue and/or their dominant language (cf. Anderson 2002: 211).[7] It may also reflect sympathy with their compatriot. Finally, as Tebble (1999) has shown, interlocutors in medical consultations can express various degrees of involvement, and the pronoun system is one of the primary channels for this. By using direct address of the patient, for instance, one of the interpreters in her study personalizes an utterance by the doctor which serves to provide reassurance, but does not contain any personal reference. By personalizing the doctor's reassurance, the interpreter conveys an even stronger sense of solidarity with the patient (1999: 191). Expressing solidarity with the patient also seems to be an important function of I(D)'s rendition in Example 5 below.

At this point in the interview, D has discovered what appears to be a miscommunication. A question by P (which was not in the script) indicates that I(D) misunderstood the diagnosis, namely that P's blood pressure is *moderately* elevated. Therefore, assuming that I(D) needs an extended explanation, D deviates from the script and addresses the interpreter, now talking *about* P.

Example 5

D19   Nej (.) altså det der (.) det her tyder på at han har det man kan kalde for et moderat forhøjet blodtryk, så han **har** et forhøjet blodtryk men det er kun lidt forhøjet.
*No (.)I mean this (.) this indicates that he has what one may call a moderately elevated blood pressure, so he **has** an elevated blood pressure but it is only slightly elevated.*

I(D) →   يعني أنت لديك أرتفاع بضغط الدم ولكن هذا ليس شيئا خطير أأ لديك قليل
أرتفاع ضغط الدم بنسبة قليلة
This means that you have a little rise of the blood pressure but it is nothing serious e:r you have a slightly elevated blood pressure with a small percentage.

Although I(D) is a consistent indirect-style interpreter, he does not use indirect or impersonal speech when relaying from D to P (a finding which is in keeping with

Cambridge's (1999: 212) description of untrained, third-person-style mediators who also tend to use the second person when relaying from D to P). The level of formality in I(D)'s rendition is reduced by his omission of D's generalized framing of the diagnosis ("what one may call") and by his substitution of the more technical *moderately* for "little." At the same time, his rendition is expanded by a reassurance ("but it is nothing serious"), which indicates his solidarity with P. However, by down-toning the importance of D's diagnosis, I(D) alters D's message in subsequent turns, whereby although P's medical condition is not serious, it has to be taken seriously because of the risk of cardiovascular diseases. Thus, the effect of I(D)'s reassurance may turn out to be harmful, which is presumably not his intention (cf. Tebble 1999 for similar cases based on authentic data with authorized interpreters).

Doctor's change of footing

In terms of participation status, D and P play the *role* of principals, although their actual status in the simulated interviews is mainly that of animators. However, they occasionally shift footing from animator to author as in Example 6 below, where D is forced to improvise. D's turn in this example is subsequent to the exchange already cited in Example 2.

> **Example 6**
> I(A) 21e Han spørger hvorhenne det er i hjertet øh at (.) at (1) at der kan ske noget.
> *He asks where it is in the heart er that (.) that (1) that something can happen.*
> D → (1) altså det med (2) / men det er / det (1) / altså der kan ske det at man kan få en blodprop som for eksempel hans / hans mor har fået, ja.
> *(1) I mean this that (2) / but it is / it (1) / I mean it may happen that one can get a blood clot like for instance his / his mother got, yes.*

D seems to be confused by the apparently unexpected question, but nevertheless tries to make sense of it and provides an answer, from her role-play position as medical expert. Her shift to the third person ("his mother") seems to be prompted by I(A)'s shift to reported speech. As D was meant to stick either to the direct form of address or — as in the context of Examples 2 and 6 — to the indefinite *one*, this shift must have been unintentional. Possibly, resuming the direct address of P in response to the interpreter's indirect speech may require more processing capacity than is available to D at this point in the discourse. Her pauses and false starts indicate that the production of a meaningful answer is proving a demanding task.

In any case, Example 6 demonstrates that interpreters' choice of address may have a profound influence on the style of address adopted by primary speakers.

Wadensjö (1997) reports similar findings in her study of an authentic interpreter-mediated police interrogation. The police officer unconsciously shifted between the direct and the indirect mode in different parts of the encounter, and Wadensjö (1997: 47) concludes, therefore, that the phenomenon "is quite obvious intuitively but should be further explored."

Patient's change of footing

Finally, we shall discuss one instance where P deviated from the script by shifting from the second to the third person. Unlike D's shift, this did not occur in response to an interpreter's use of indirect speech, but in response to a rendition which appears to be inconsistent with information given earlier in the discourse, as illustrated in Example 7.

The extract starts with D's explanation of the term *risk factor*, following I(C)'s request for clarification.

> **Example 7**
> D23 Men altså (xxx) for at illustrere det så kan jeg sige at (.) at hvis for eksempel din familie + hvis der i din familie er nogle der har forhøjet blodtryk eller har **haft** forhøjet blodtryk eller er død af en blodprop i hjertet. Det er en risikofaktor.
> *But I mean (xxx) to illustrate it I can say that (.) that if for example your family + if there in your family are some who have elevated blood pressure or have **had** elevated blood pressure or have died of a blood clot in the heart. That is a risk factor.*
>
> Ic. لو في حد في عائلتك أ مات أو حصلت لو أزمة أأ بسبب الضغط أرتفاع ضغط الدم أو إنسداد شرايين الألب ده التي بتسمح ممكن أنت يجيلك مرض ضغط الدم
> *If there is anybody in your family er who died or had a crisis e:r because of a rise of the blood pressure or blocked arteries in the heart this allows that it becomes possible that you get the blood pressure disease.*
>
> Ic. أرتفاع ضغط الدم
> *Rise of blood pressure.*
>
> P → ضغط الدم مرض؟ هي قالت مش مرض.
> *Blood pressure disease? She said [it was] not [a] disease.*
>
> I(C) → Du sagde / (1) er (1) er (2) højt blodtryk en sygdom? Du sagde at det ikke var.
> *You said / (1) is (1) is (2) high blood pressure a disease? You said that it was not.*

D   <u>(xxx) jeg har hele tiden sagt</u> og det holder jeg fast i at højt blodtryk er ikke en sygdom som sådan.
         <u>(xxx) I have been saying all the time</u> and I stick to this that high blood pressure is not a disease as such.

Ic.   ضغط الدم مش مرض بحد ذاتو بالشكل ده
         Blood pressure is not a disease in itself as such.

P   هي لسه آيله أنه مرض
         She just said that it was a disease.

I(C) →   Du har lige sagt at det er en sygdom.
         You just said that it is a disease.

D   Nej det har jeg ikke (griner).
         No I have not (laughs).

I(C)'s rendition of D's first utterance is reduced — she omits D's reference to prior meta-talk ("to illustrate it I can say that") and her false start. It also includes several expansions — among others, I(C) introduces an (erroneous) example of a risk factor, "blood pressure disease." P reacts by an echoic question ("blood pressure disease?"), having been told a few minutes earlier that high blood pressure is *not* a disease. Presumably, he failed to hear I(C)'s immediate self-correction, because of the overlap.

I(C)'s handling of P's protest results in miscommunication. She turns P's question into a standard request for information, thereby altering its pragmatic meaning and disclaiming responsibility for the incorrect expansion she herself introduced in her rendition of D's explanation. She then continues her turn by providing a substituted rendition of P's indirect speech, shifting to the second person *you*, which is her usual style of interpreting. By this shift, I(C) assumes the role of non-person and creates the impression that D, and not herself, was the intended addressee of P's critical remark.

As a result, D apparently perceives I(C)'s utterance as an interpreter request for clarification instead of seeing it as a rendition. Moreover, D seems to perceive the utterance as inappropriate, questioning her professionalism, presumably due to I(C)'s repetition of "you said." The exchange then develops into an argument, with I(C) again adopting the technique of relaying P's second turn in the extract, instead of engaging in explicit coordinating. Thus, I(C) fails to take responsibility for the miscommunication just as she fails to clarify the participation framework (cf. Wadensjö 1999). If she had made a shift to *I* meaning *self*, she could have assumed responsibility and presumably cleared up the miscommunication. I(C) introduces this shift four times elsewhere in the interview in order to solve interactional problems, but for some reason omits it here. At this point in the interaction, she may have forgotten who said what, and also seems to have trouble concentrating on a correct rendering of D's "elevated blood pressure" for the second time in

Example 7. Thus, I(C)'s reduced rendition does not make sense ("Blood pressure is not a disease in itself") — and may indicate her lack of familiarity with this medical concept.

Factors affecting the superiority of the direct style

As demonstrated in Example 7, the direct style of interpreting may not be an adequate way of managing miscommunication. Occasionally, shifts to *I* meaning *self* or to indirect address may be necessary in order to clarify the authorship of particular utterances. Thus, dependent on special contexts, other modes of address may appear to be superior to the direct style.

The data show that the superiority of the direct style may be affected by yet another factor, namely the extent of one-language talk between the interpreter and one of the primary parties. This may disturb the illusion of directness of communication between the primary parties, which is the main rationale behind the direct style of interpreting (cf. Wadensjö 1997: 49).

One-language talk is often triggered by *non-renditions*, i.e. — as referred to previously — interpreters' initiatives or responses which do not correspond to a prior 'original'. In our data, almost all non-renditions are responses to the prior speaker in the form of requests for clarification of medical terms. These responses "tend to produce one-language sequences between the DI [dialogue interpreter] and the primary party involved, thus temporarily excluding the other PP [primary party] from the conversation" Wadensjö (1992: 73).

In what follows, an attempt is made to give a rough idea of the extent of one-language talk in each of the four interviews, by means of the overviews in Tables 4 and 5.

Table 4 shows which expressions triggered non-renditions (and produced one-language sequences) involving which interpreter (indicated by capital letters following the terms).

Most requests for clarification concerned common-language medical expressions. As mentioned previously, there were no specialized medical terms, i.e. Latin- or Greek-based ones, in the script, either in Danish or in Arabic. Common-language medical terms and "hybrid" terms such as *moderately* elevated blood pressure, have been referred to as "semi-professional medical expressions" (Löning & Rehbein 1995, quoted in Meyer 2001: 90). Doctors tend to prefer them when talking with patients because they believe that these terms are more readily comprehensible (Rehbein 1985; Meyer 2001).

The seemingly user-friendly terminology does not help much if the patient — or the untrained interpreter — lacks knowledge of the medical concept in question

Table 4. Non-rendition triggers

Semi-professional medical terms		Non-medical Latin-/Greek-based terms	
نزيف في الأنف *(nosebleed)*	B	control *(control)*	C
blodtryk *(blood pressure)*	B	risikofaktorer *(risk factors)*	B, C
جلطة دموية في القلب *(blood clot in the heart)*	B, C	symptomer *(symptoms)*	C
nedre blodtryk *(lower blood pressure)*	D	tendens *(tendency)*	B
moderat forhøjet blodtryk *(moderately elevated blood pressure)*	B, C		
højt blodtryk *(high blood pressure)*	C		
hjerte-kar-sygdomme *(heart and [blood] vessel diseases)*	B, C, D		

(Rehbein 1985; Meyer 2001; Bührig & Meyer 2004). Thus semi-professional terminology is accessible only to lay persons with a certain educational background, i.e. at least upper secondary school level (Shuy 1976; referred to in Rehbein 1985: 402). It is not surprising then that I(A), whose educational background meets this requirement, is not represented in Table 4 at all. It is not clear, however, why I(C), who has a similar background, asks for clarification many times.

Apart from medical terms, Table 4 contains some non-medical expressions that are fairly frequent in everyday Danish. However, as they are Latin- or Greek-based, they turned out to be unknown to two of the Arabic interpreters and therefore trigger non-renditions.

Table 4 comprises only items that prompted explicit non-rendition turns. It does not capture plain wrong renditions which remained without comment, nor reduced renditions, e.g. I(A): "heart diseases" instead of "cardiovascular diseases," nor substituted renditions functioning as compensating strategies (cf. Bührig & Meyer 2004), e.g. I(D): "diabetes and other things" instead of "diabetes and kidney diseases." It was a surprise for the testers/researchers to find that so many common medical expressions as well as non-medical expressions proved to be a challenge for the interpreters.

Table 5 shows that the extent of one-language talk (expressed as the number of non-rendition triggers) affected the length of the interviews quite substantially.

It is striking that the same role play takes only 12 minutes with I(A), but 16 minutes with I(C). If it may be assumed that the smooth flow of the interpreted

Table 5. Number of non-rendition triggers and length of interview

Interpreter	Style	Number of triggers	Length of interview
A	direct	0	12 min.
D	indirect	2	14 min.
B	indirect	7	15 min.
C	direct	7	16 min.

interviews can be expressed in terms of the length of the encounter, then the direct-style interpreter A performed best. (With one exception, not captured in Tables 4 and 5, there were no interruptions.) By contrast, the other direct-style interpreter, C, performed worst. Moreover, together with B, she had the highest score of interruptions.

There is thus no obvious connection between the interpreter's use of the direct style and the smoothness of the interview. Rather, the latter seems to be related to the interpreters' educational background, language proficiency and experience. For instance, the indirect-style interpreter B, whose mother tongue is Kurdish and whose command of Arabic and Danish is insufficient, causes the doctor to intervene, repeat and explain almost constantly, with the interpreter as intended addressee. Consequently, the doctor needs to refer to the patient in the third person 12 times (cf. Table 3). As regards I(C), her many clarification turns and other non-renditions are presumably due to her lack of experience. The proportion of one-language talk excluding one or the other of the primary parties from the exchange is thus the main factor affecting the quasi-directness of communication in our data.

Conclusion

Our study of four untrained interpreters' use of direct vs. indirect styles of address shows that one particular word triggered the same kind of shift, regardless of whether the interpreters preferred the direct or the indirect style: All four interpreters changed the doctor's indefinite *one* into the second person singular *you*, thereby "personalizing" (Tebble 1999) the doctor's speech.

Personalizing utterances is not conditioned by differences between the languages involved in the present study. Consequently, it may be an indication of the interpreters' solidarity with the patient, their rapport with their fellow compatriot, or their identification with the speaker of their mother tongue and/or dominant language. This personalizing of utterances is used not only by the untrained interpreters in our study, but also by trained professionals (Tebble 1999) and thus seems to be an obvious field for further study — particularly in view of the fact that it may counteract healthcare providers' communicative purposes.

All other types of interpreters' pronoun shifts in the data seemed to indicate distance and reservation, or to function as compensating strategies, when interactional problems were caused by the interpreters' lack of familiarity with medical terminology.

The primary participants both shifted to indirect speech although they were supposed to address each other directly, as per the script. Their shifts occurred primarily in response to an interpreter's request for repetition or clarification, but also in response to incorrect renditions. Finally, some shifts seem to have been intuitive, prompted by an interpreter's change of footing, in the form of a shift to reported speech.

As regards the superiority of the direct mode of interpreting, the data show that it can be affected in two ways. Firstly, reported speech can be necessary in cases where the referent of the *I* meaning *other*, or the direct address *you* is ambiguous. Thus, the direct mode sometimes has to be complemented, by switching either to the third person or to the *I* meaning *self*, in order to avoid miscommunication. Secondly, the quasi-directness of communication between the monolingual parties can be reduced considerably by repeated one-language talk triggered by problems with medical terminology and/or lack of familiarity with medical concepts. The data show that an indirect-style interpreter with more relevant knowledge and experience than a direct-style interpreter may be more able to ensure smoothness of communication.

The extent to which deficiencies in the interpreters' medical knowledge base caused interactional problems in three of the four interviews was a surprise to the testers. Likewise, the researchers did not expect the amount of misinformation and loss of information relating to the medical context that was revealed in the transcriptions. As the non-Arabic-speaking doctor in the role play is in a position similar to that of most professional healthcare providers who work with interpreters in Denmark, there is reason to believe that doctors in authentic situations are not aware of the extent of the problem either. Thus, it seems that, in order to minimize serious miscommunication in interpreter-mediated medical encounters, it is necessary not only to test untrained community interpreters, but also to offer awareness-raising seminars for healthcare providers. Finally, there also seems to be very good reason to point out the importance of training the untrained interpreters, specifically in specialized terminology.

Acknowledgement

We are grateful to Omar Dhahir, PhD. Without his help and commitment, this study would not have been possible.

Notes

1. In the Arabic part of the data, direct or indirect reference can be indicated by verb morphemes alone.

2. A certified community interpreter (Danish *Statsprøvet tolk*) has completed a two-year part-time university-level programme in Danish and one other language at the Copenhagen Business School. The programme covers social, medical and legal interpreting.

3. We apply Wadensjö's (1997: 48) definition of a turn as "a sequence in which one person is speaking without interruption. It commences when this person starts talking and ends when speech stops. Hence, when two people speak at the same time, two turns occur simultaneously (or partly simultaneously)." As regards the number of turns in the script, these were not always followed closely during the tests, because long turns were sometimes split into several shorter ones if this was considered necessary by the testers or was asked for by the interpreters.

4. That this is a reasonable assumption appears from one occasion in the role play where I(C) treats the beginning of a summarized rendition in reported speech as a false start ("he had / I had a handkerchief in my pocket").

5. Similar pronoun shifts from second person singular to second person plural are made by Wadensjö's (1998b: 116–117) interpreters when relaying from Swedish to Russian.

6. As regards exceptions from I(B)'s indirect style, the data do not reveal any particular function of his two shifts to *I* meaning other (whereas one shift to *I* meaning *self* — *His mother is dead in the way I told [you]*"– is designed to avoid specific reference to the concept of *blood clot in the heart* which had caused I(B) to ask for clarification in the previous context).

7. Anderson speaks about the interpreter's identification with the *monolingual* speaker of his/her mother tongue. The patient in our study is of course not monolingual, but as this is normally the case, the interpreters may have followed their usual linguistic behaviour in the test situation.

References

Adams, C., Corsellis, A. & Harmer, A. (1995). *Basic handbook for trainers of public service interpreters*. London: Institute of Linguists.
Anderson, R. B. W. (1976/2002). Perspectives on the role of interpreter. In F. Pöchhacker & M. Shlesinger (Eds.), *The interpreting studies reader*. London/New York: Routledge, 209–217.
Baaring, I. (2001). *Tolkning — hvor og hvordan?* Frederiksberg: Samfundslitteratur.

Bot, H. (2003). The myth of the uninvolved interpreter interpreting in mental health and the development of a three-person psychology. In L. Brunette, G. Bastin, I. Hemlin & H. Clarke (Eds.), *The critical link 3. Interpreters in the community. Selected papers from the Third International Conference on Interpreting in Legal, Health and Social Service Settings*, Montreal 22–26 May 2001. Amsterdam/Philadelphia: John Benjamins, 27–35.

Bührig, K. & Meyer, B. (2004). Ad hoc-interpreting and the achievement of communicative purposes in specific kinds of doctor-patient discourse. In *Working Papers in Multilingualism* 57, Universität Hamburg.

Cambridge, J. (1999). Information loss in bilingual medical interviews through an untrained interpreter. *The Translator* 5 (2), 201–219.

Dansk Flygtningehjælp (2001). *Flygtningehjælpens Tolkeservice Vest. Information og vejledning for tilkaldetolke.*

Domstolsstyrelsen (2003). *Rapport om tolkebistand i retssager.* Appendix 4, Guidelines for court interpreting. Copenhagen.

Driesen, C. (2002). Gerichtsdolmetschen — Praxis und Problematik. In J. Best & S. Kalina (Eds.), *Übersetzen und Dolmetschen: Eine Orientierungshilfe.* Tübingen/Basel: Francke, 299–306.

Galal, L. P. & Galal, E. (1999). *Goddag mand, økseskaft.* Copenhagen: Mellemfolkeligt Samvirke.

Gentile, A., Ozolins, U. & Vasilakakos, M. (1996). *Liaison interpreting: A handbook.* Melbourne: Melbourne University Press.

Gill, S. & Kristensen, S. D. (no year). Forhøjet blodtryk (hypertension). *NetDoktor.* http://www.netdoktor.dk/sygdomme/fakta/hypertension.htm (accessed 23 July 2004).

Goffman, E. (1981). *Forms of talk.* Oxford: Blackwell.

Hale, S. B. (2004). *The discourse of court interpreting: Discourse practices of the law, the witness and the interpreter.* Amsterdam/Philadelphia: John Benjamins.

Harris, B. (1990). Norms in interpretation. *Target* 2 (1), 115–119.

Knapp, K. & Knapp-Potthoff, A. (1985). Sprachmittlertätigkeit in interkultureller Kommunikation. In J. Rehbein (Ed.), *Interkulturelle Kommunikation.* Tübingen: Narr, 450–463.

Lings, K. K. (1988). *Dynamisk tolkning.* Herning: Special-pædagogisk forlag.

Löning, P. & Rehbein, J. (1995). Sprachliche Verständigungsprozesse in der Arzt-Patienten-Kommunikation. Linguistische Untersuchungen von Gesprächen in der Facharzt-Praxis. *Arbeiten zur Mehrsprachigkeit* 54. Universität Hamburg, Germanisches Seminar.

Mason, I. (1999). Introduction. *The Translator* 5 (2), Special issue, 147–160.

Meyer, B. (2001). How untrained interpreters handle medical terms. In I. Mason (Ed.), *Triadic exchanges: Studies in dialogue interpreting.* Manchester/Northampton, MA: St. Jerome, 87–106.

Meyer, B. (2002). Untersuchungen zu den Aufgaben des interkulturellen Mittelns. In J. Best & S. Kalina (Eds.), *Übersetzen und Dolmetschen: Eine Orientierungshilfe.* Tübingen/Basel: Francke, 51–59.

Metzger, M. (1999). *Sign language interpreting: Deconstructing the myth of neutrality.* Washington, DC: Gallaudet University Press.

Niska, H. (1999). Status quaestionis: Community interpreting in Sweden. In M. Erasmus (Ed.), *Liaison interpreting in the community.* Pretoria: van Schaik, 138–142.

Phelan, M. (2001). *The interpreter's resource.* Clevedon/Buffalo/Toronto/Sydney: Multilingual Matters.

Pöchhacker, F. (2004). *Introducing interpreting studies.* London/New York: Routledge.

Razban, M. (2003). An interpreter's perspective. In R. Tribe & H. Raval (Eds.), *Working with interpreters in mental health*. Hove/New York: Brunner-Routledge, 92–98.

Rehbein, J. (1985). Medizinische Beratung türkischer Eltern. In J. Rehbein (Ed.), *Interkulturelle Kommunikation*. Tübingen: Narr, 349–419.

Shackman, J. (1984). *The right to be understood*. Cambridge: National Extension College.

Shlesinger, M. (1991). Interpreter latitude vs. due process: Simultaneous and consecutive interpretation in multilingual trials. In S. Tirkkonen-Condit (Ed.), *Empirical research in translation and intercultural studies*. Selected papers from the TRANSIF seminar, Savonlinna 1988. Tübingen: Narr, 147–155.

Shuy, R. W. (1976). The medical interview. Problems in communication. *Primary Care* 3, 365–386.

Tebble, H. (1999). The tenor of consultant physicians. *The Translator* 5 (2), 179–200.

Wadensjö, C. (1992). *Interpreting as interaction. On dialogue interpreting in immigration hearings and medical encounters*. Linköping University.

Wadensjö, C. (1993). Dialogue interpreting and shared knowledge. In Y. Gambier & J. Tommola (Eds.), *Translation and knowledge*. Proceedings of the Fourth Scandinavian Symposium on Translation Theory, Turku 4–6 June 1992. Turku: University of Turku, Centre for Translation and Interpreting, 101–113.

Wadensjö, C. (1997). Recycled information as a questioning strategy: Pitfalls in interpreter-mediated talk. In S. E. Carr, R. Roberts, A. Dufour & D. Stein (Eds.), *The critical link: Interpreters in the community*. Amsterdam/Philadelphia: John Benjamins, 35–52.

Wadensjö, C. (1998a). Community interpreting. In M. Baker (Ed.), *Routledge encyclopaedia of translation studies*. London/New York: Routledge, 33–37.

Wadensjö, C. (1998b). *Interpreting as interaction*. London/New York: Longman.

Wadensjö, C. (1999). Telephone interpreting and the synchronization of talk. *The Translator* 5 (2), 247–264.

Dialogue interpreting as a specific case of reported speech

Hanneke Bot

De Gelderse Roos, Wolfheze, The Netherlands

This paper reports on what is often referred to as "translating in the first person" or retaining the perspective of person as an aspect of consecutive interpreting that generates attention whenever the quality of interpreting is being considered. The study draws on six videotaped interpreter-mediated psychotherapy sessions and constitutes part of a PhD research project (described in Bot 2005) on the communication processes in interpreter-mediated psychotherapeutic dialogue. The study shows it is possible to distinguish between two types of changes in the perspective of person: the addition of a reporting verb (e.g. "he says"), generally at the beginning of a rendition, and a change in personal pronoun (usually from "I" into "he" or "she") in what follows. All three of the interpreters in the data sample introduce these two types of changes, at different frequencies and for various reasons. The findings show that the addition of a reporting verb not only serves to indicate who is speaking, but also plays a role in the organization of turn-transfer. They also suggest that changes in the perspective of person are less of a problem than generally assumed. Although such shifts do serve to indicate the specific position of the interpreter as intermediary between therapist and patient, this does not seem to alienate therapist and patient, but merely recognizes the interactive reality of this type of talk.

1. Introduction

I began my research into the communication processes in interpreter-mediated psychotherapeutic dialogue by interviewing therapists, patients and interpreters, and asking them what factors they believed to be important in enabling interpreter-mediated therapy to proceed well. These factors were then constructed into models using a structured-brainstorm procedure (concept mapping). The second part of the research comprised the analysis of six video-recorded interpreter-mediated psychotherapy sessions, which were kept as "true to nature" as possible to ensure ecological validity. All of the participants were aware that they were being recorded and had consented to this procedure, but the researcher did not intervene in the proceedings in any other way. Two consecutive sessions of three groups were recorded, each consisting of a therapist, a patient and an interpreter. These groups are referred to here as Groups One, Two and Three. Thus, reference is made, for example, to Interpreter One working for Therapist One and Patient One, etc.

The recordings were made at three state-recognized mental-health institutions in the Netherlands. The therapists were experienced state-certified therapists who had specialized in treating asylum seekers and refugees, and had ample experience working with interpreters. The interpreters were all employed by the Dutch Interpreter and Translation Center, a government-funded organization providing interpreter services to the social sector. They were professionals, in the sense that they made a living by interpreting, subscribed to a code of conduct and had committed themselves to maintaining confidentiality. Most of them had not undergone official training in interpreting, but had had to pass exams (language proficiency in both languages, general knowledge of the countries involved, a memory test and role plays) to be included in the Center's roster of interpreters. The three interpreters had Dari and Persian as their mother tongues and Dutch as their second language. The therapists had been requested to select an interpreter with whom they had worked frequently, who they felt was a "good interpreter" and with whom they "cooperated well." The patients were asylum seekers who had been diagnosed with Post-Traumatic Stress Disorder, and the sessions recorded were from the middle phase of their treatment. They spoke Dari and Persian, languages spoken in Iran and Afghanistan. Throughout this article, the term "primary speaker" will be used to refer to the therapist and the patient. These "primary speakers" take ("primary") turns, and these are rendered by the interpreter.

One of the issues encountered during the study was that of "*directe vertaling*" (literally, direct translation):[1] Interpreters are instructed by the Interpreter Center to provide a "direct translation" of what the primary speakers say, which means, among other things, that they should not change the perspective of person. I have noticed that users of interpreter services believe the interpretation to be good when they note that interpreters render the translation in the first person, and seem to treat the retention of the perspective of person as *the* sign of professionalism.

After the material had been transcribed and translated, my initial impression was that the interpreters frequently violated this "rule of direct translation." Upon closer examination, however, it was found that this impression was only partially correct — most often the interpreters added "he says" at the beginning of a rendition, but continued with a direct translation.

In this article, interpreter renditions and the issue of "direct translation" are related to the concepts of reported speech as constructed dialogue (Tannen 1989), perspective and the related concept of mental space (Fauconnier 1985; Sanders 1994), and the effects of changes in the perspective of person in the interpreted utterances of therapist and patient in the six sessions are discussed. The findings indicate that each interpreter has his/her own style of dealing with the perspective of person. Most deviations from direct translation, as defined above, take the form of "direct reported speech." The article concludes with the formulation of a new approach to the issue of perspective of person in interpreter-mediated dialogue.

The study on which this paper is based was conducted in what Pöchhacker (2004) calls the dialogic-interactive paradigm of interpreting, introduced by Wadensjö (1998) and followed by Roy (2000), among others. Although not discussed at length in the current paper, this approach is discussed in Bot (2005), which is based on my doctoral dissertation.

2.   Reported speech

"Reported speech" is the term commonly used to report something that was said in the past. Tannen (1989: 98) writes about reported speech in a manner that may be helpful in understanding the character of interpreter-mediated dialogue. She states that reported speech not only comes in the generally assumed forms of direct (he said: "I'll come") and indirect reported speech (he said that he would come), but also in a multitude of other forms. Tannen further argues that the term "reported speech" is in fact misleading, as it gives the impression that words repeated in a different context may remain untransformed. She goes on to say that reported speech is creatively constructed by a current speaker in a current situation: "uttering dialogue in conversation is as much a creative act as the creation of dialogue in fiction and drama" (p. 101).

The task of interpreters is commonly described as "to translate what a speaker just said into another language." In the Netherlands, interpreters are instructed, mainly through their Code of Conduct, to *translate directly*, i.e. without changing the perspective of person, what the speakers just said. This leads to an even more direct form of reporting than the one Tannen dubbed "direct reported speech." When the therapist says "I have a headache," the interpreter says "I have a headache," though in a different language, without the addition of "he said" as in Tannen's example of "direct reported speech." It is possible to say that interpreters are instructed to *repeat* speech. The guideline assumes that both primary speakers know the rules of the game and understand that these are the words of the primary speaker and not utterances made at the interpreters' initiative. It further assumes that it is possible to "repeat" the original words in a different language.

2.1 Who is responsible?

Tannen introduces different attitudes toward reported speech that are interesting in the context of dialogue interpreting, and notes that in the United States, it is "folk knowledge" that when someone reports criticism, this criticism is understood to come not from the last speaker, but from the person who was quoted. She writes that "any anger and hurt felt in response to reported criticism is, for Americans at least, typically directed toward the quoted source rather than the speaker who conveys the criticism. (In contrast, according to an Arab proverb, 'the one who repeats an insult is the one who is insulting you'" (pp. 105–106)). Tannen therefore calls the first attitude the "American" way of dealing with reported speech, the second one the "Arabic" way. Although equating attitudes towards indirect speech with ethnic characteristics is unfortunate, the distinction Tannen makes is interesting when taken in the context of interpreting. The emphasis on direct translation in interpreter education and job description assumes an "American" attitude towards reported speech. Tannen continues to say that criticism uttered in a context in which the criticized person is not present is fundamentally different from criticism uttered in the presence of that person. Assuming that a "reporting person" is not responsible for the reported words means that the conveyor is seen as an "inert vessel" transmitting information and that the sole responsibility for this information lies with the quoted party. This is an attitude that reflects "the pervasive American attitude toward language and communication that [is known] as the conduit metaphor, the misconception of communication as merely a matter of exchanging information, language being a neutral conduit" (p. 109). Instead, Tannen argues that what has been called "reported speech" is in fact "constructed dialogue" in which speakers choose whether or not to report (parts of) what others said earlier and in a different context. This implies they can be held responsible for what they report; i.e. the "Arabic" attitude, which may better be referred to as the "responsible messenger" approach.

3. Perspective and mental space theory

The term perspective refers to a complex concept describing the viewpoint from which speakers or writers speak or write. Related to this concept is the idea of "mental spaces." Sanders (1994) supposes that these concepts, coined by Fauconnier (1985) and used in the analysis of written texts, are not significantly different in spoken language.

3.1 Perspective

The production and understanding of perspectivized information is required for social interaction through language (Sanders 1994: 3). "Texts," in fact, all communication, "can be misunderstood completely if one fails to understand from which perspective statements are presented" (p. 14). Sanders describes the ability to understand perspectivized information and to use different perspectives as a complex skill that develops gradually. Children are not yet equipped to take another person's point of view until the age of 3–4. Then, gradually, when egocentric tendencies decrease, language becomes more interactional, and children become aware of other people's perspectives and adapt their language to them. Perspective is described as a complex phenomenon in monolingual communication. Understanding whose perspective is used and whose point of view is represented in discourse requires mature language and communication skills.

Sanders distinguishes three aspects of perspective: "worldview," "subjective point of view" and "vantage point." **Worldview** is the point of view from which one perceives and presents the world, consisting of "a coherent world of beliefs and attitudes with respect to perceptions of the 'other' and 'self' as well as the perception of 'the problem' and proposed solutions to this 'problem'" (Sanders 1994: 6).

Subjective point of view implies that the speaker is not necessarily the person whose perspective is represented. The speaker may choose to represent someone else's worldview or vantage point. In the sessions recorded for this study, the primary speakers generally speak for themselves: They use their own worldview and refer to themselves as "I." However, it occasionally happens that the primary speakers report other people's words. Typically, therapists repeat the words of the patient, and patients may report the words of their spouses, children or lawyers. The primary speakers then use someone else's worldview and vantage point for a while; i.e. they report speech. This immediately points to a problem that might manifest itself in interpreter-mediated talk: in interpreter renditions, this pattern becomes "reported speech within reported speech."

Vantage point refers to deixis and is described by Sanders as "the 'camera angle' from which a scene is presented." It involves time, place and person indicators. As far as "person" is concerned, it defines the "I," "you" and "s/he" about which the interlocutors are speaking. During the interaction, the vantage point may change, meaning that the "I," the "you" and "s/he" do not have to refer to the same persons throughout a verbal exchange or throughout a text. In interpreter-mediated talk, the indicator of person is particularly interesting as it refers directly to the issue of "who is talking" and to the different attitudes towards "reported speech". It is therefore most susceptible to changes by interpreters, as they may want to indicate that the words they speak do not come from them. Paradoxically, then, when we look at interpreter renditions as text, a change of perspective compared to the primary text means a change of vantage point, but when we look at their renditions as an interactive phenomenon, the vantage point is changed to emphasize that the subjective point of view still belongs to the primary speaker. The present article focuses on the "vantage point" aspect and specifically on that of "person".

3.2 Mental space theory

In mental space theory it is assumed that understanding a narrative involves the creation of a mental world in which "domains" or *mental spaces* are formed (Fauconnier 1985; Sanders 1994). A mental space can be understood as representing a specific perspective, within which "validity" and "truth" are defined as subjective concepts. In narration, as in dialogue, several perspectives can be intertwined. Readers and listeners create mental spaces and attribute the information they receive to these spaces. "A mental space is always set up subordinate of a 'parent space.' The outermost parent space is that of the speaker's reality and is called the 'base space'" (Sanders 1994: 17–18).

The basic idea of mental space theory is "the claim that sentences are partial instructions for building, connecting and structuring domains in discourse" (1994: 17). Narrators and speakers use linguistic devices to create the various mental spaces. Those devices which serve to establish a (sub)space are called "spacebuilders," which "mark the material in the embedded space as restricted to a particular temporal, spatial, hypothetical or counterfactual situation or to a particular (subjective) belief or perspective" (1994: 18). Mental spaces are set up not only by explicit space builders, but also by "more indirect grammatical means (such as shifts in tense or mood) and also by non-linguistic pragmatic, cultural and contextual factors" (1994: 22). In spoken language, prosodic and non-verbal devices such as gesture and gaze can be used as space builders as well.

"Perspective" and "mental space" are related dialectically. Perspective helps create mental spaces, while mental space theory offers a descriptive and explanatory model for the use and existence of perspective in discourse.

4.   Interpreters: Translation machines or interacting persons?

The "American" attitude to reported speech as described by Tannen (1989) refers to the "reporter" as an inert vessel. In dialogue interpreting, this concept is reflected in what is sometimes referred to as the conduit model or the translation-machine model, in which the interpreter is seen as a "non-person," a mere conveyor of messages in a different language. This conceptualization is contrasted here with an interactive model of interpreting, in which interpreters are viewed as active participants in the dialogue, whose main task is to translate the words of the primary speakers. In such an interactive model, interpreters may be concerned about being seen as responsible for the words they translate, as responsible messengers. This differentiation in the interpreter's role is similar to the one between interpreting as text or as interaction, as discussed extensively by Wadensjö (1998).

As stated above, an initial examination of the transcripts reveals that interpreters frequently stray from direct translation style as prescribed by the Interpreter Center. Various reasons suggest themselves:

First, interpreters are obviously not translation machines. They come to the task with feelings, opinions, memories and preconceptions about psychotherapy and about the participants' roles in the psychotherapeutic setting. They may feel the need to distance themselves from the words they translate and may have doubts regarding the primary speakers' understanding of their role. This is where the concepts of "reported speech," "perspective" and "mental space" enter the world of interpreter-mediated dialogue. When interpreter-mediated dialogue is viewed in terms of "reported speech," the issue of mental space representation and space building becomes a complex aspect of the task. Changes in perspective may very well lead to changes in the mental spaces that are elucidated, i.e. they may lead to the attribution of "content" to other spaces than those intended by the primary speakers.

Use of the direct form *is* an issue for interpreters and users of interpreting services alike. The users generally see the addition of "he says" and/or a shift into the third person as a lack of professionalism on the part of the interpreter. It is not surprising that users of interpreting services relate to this issue, as it is something that is readily noticed, while other changes introduced by interpreters to the words of primary speakers are not as easily noticed and can only be observed through "circumstantial evidence," if at all.

The importance of this issue for interpreters can be seen, for example, in the July–August 2002 discussions conducted on the NCIHC-list, the online discussion group of the U.S. National Council on Interpreting in Health Care. In the exchange of views, it emerged that some participants in the discussion favored the direct form, as it kept the original intact, while others believed it was unnecessary and that it only served to emphasize the myth of the translation machine. In her study of interpreting for the Truth and Reconciliation Committee in South Africa, Wallmach (2002) stresses that the closeness between interpreter and speaker caused by using the "I" form may take an emotional toll (a subject that is mentioned on the NCIHC-list but is not presented as problematic.) The paradox is that while interpreters add the "s/he says" formulation to stress their role as "mere conveyor of the message," the very addition is in itself a deviation from the strict conveyor model.

One of the interpreters recorded almost always renders the words of the patient through a direct translation, using the pronoun "I," but adds "he says" when interpreting the words of the therapist, thus making it "direct reported speech." When asked about this tendency, the interpreter explained: "I know the therapist understands the procedure, he understands that these words are not mine, but the patient's. I'm not sure though that the patient understands this, and I want to make clear to him that these are the words of the therapist." In other words, this interpreter ascribes the "inert vessel" attitude to the therapist and the "responsible messenger" attitude to the patient.

The other two interpreters frequently add "he says," to the words of both the therapist and the patient, but fail to offer a clear explanation for their behaviour. They say it is "just natural" to add "s/he says," which seems to imply that they equate interpreter-mediated dialogue with "ordinary" conversation, in which they report what was said by another person. The addition of a "s/he says" formulation by the interpreter does not immediately imply that the interpreter has changed the perspective of the original text in the following rendition. It does however emphasize that the interpreters are not using their own words. By choosing this formulation, interpreters assign themselves a place of their own as interactive participants in the dialogue. The "s/he says" formulation when starting a rendition functions as an explicit space builder. It indicates that the material in the interpreted version is restricted to a particular subjective perspective (that of the preceding primary speaker) and should be seen as belonging to the base space of that speaker.

5.   Changes in perspective of person

The focus of the current study is the relationship between the perspective of person in the utterance of the primary speaker and the perspective in its rendition by the interpreter. (The reasons for the primary speaker's choice of perspective are not the focus of the present study, although it might be worthy of further research.)

5.1 Taxonomy of change in perspective

Let us first relate briefly to the unit of analysis selected for study. In written narrative, perspective is studied in sentences or in text parts. In interpreter-mediated interaction, the obvious unit of analysis is the turn. It has clear boundaries, and forms the structural backbone of the dialogue. Turns vary in length. In the material examined here, some consist of only one word or a few words, while others are made up of several sentences and over two hundred words. As we are dealing with spoken language, it is sometimes easier to distinguish different bits of information within a turn than to identify separate sentences. The sequence in which the bits of information are presented in the original is not always the same in the rendition. As a result, it is difficult to compare the primary turn and its rendition at the sub-turn level. A decision was therefore made to analyze changes of perspective at the turn level; i.e. a complete turn of a primary speaker is compared with the immediately following turn of the interpreter.

Haarhuis (2003) raises two key questions, which form the basis of a taxonomy of changes in perspective of person in interpreter-mediated talk:

1. Does the interpreter use a **reporting verb**, i.e. does s/he add "s/he says" or a similar marker — to the words s/he translates? This strategy is referred to as a "*representation form*" whereas a translation without reporting verb is referred to as a "*translation form.*"
2. Does the interpreter use the same **perspective of person** as the primary speaker? For example: when the primary speaker says "I went to school," does the interpreter say "I went to school" (the "*direct*" perspective) or does s/he change the perspective to "he went to school" (the "*indirect*" perspective). Most often, the perspective of person changes from first person to third. In rare instances there are other changes in the perspective as well.

The answer to these two questions leads to a distinction among four main strategies of perspective change:

Table 1. Taxonomy of change of perspective of person (original utterance: "I went to school")

Perspective / Reporting verb	Perspective unchanged	Perspective changed
Yes	1.Direct representation *he says I went to school*	2. Indirect representation *he says (that) he went to school*
No	3. Direct translation *I went to school*	4. Indirect translation *he went to school*

The direct representation is what Tannen (1989) calls "direct reported speech," while indirect representation is equivalent to "indirect reported speech." The following are examples of these four strategies identified in the material examined in the current study:

1. Direct representation[2]
Turn 4:Th: 093[3]

> T   ik begin het nu te begrijpen
> *I start it now to understand*
> I   mīgūyand, man al'ān tāze rāsteš rā bekhāhīd motawajjeh šodam
> *he says, I it now just to be honest have understood*

The interpreter uses a reporting verb ("he says") to indicate that the following words were uttered by the therapist, after which he renders the words of the therapist directly; the "he says" formulation is here used as an explicit space builder.

The following example is also a direct representation, but is different from the preceding one.

Turn 2:Th: 007

> T   ja, en dat is anders, u bent meer vermoeid dan normaal, eigenlijk
> *yes, and that is different, you are more tired than usual, so to say*
> I   mīgūyand, pas šomā khastetar hastīd az hālat-e 'ādî?
> *he says, than you are more tired than in the usual situation?*

The therapist addresses the patient with "you." The interpreter translates the therapist's words using the same perspective of person, "you," and adds "he says" at the beginning of his turn as a space builder. The interpreter thus uses a representation form and a direct perspective. In the first example, the interpreter could have changed the utterance in "*he said he it now just to be honest has understood,*" thus making it an indirect representation without confusing the issue of who actually understood. In this second example, the therapist uses the second person, but the interpreter cannot change the personal pronoun without changing the entire meaning of the utterance. These two examples present renditions as *direct reported speech*.

Apart from the function of explicit space builder, a reporting verb also has a function in the turn transfer from the primary speaker to the interpreter. When the interpreter wants to take her/his turn with a brief overlap from the previous speaker, the use of "s/he says" serves as a turn-entry device (Streeck & Hartge 1992) to indicate the desire for turn transfer without any information loss due to overlapping talk.

2.   Indirect representation
Turn 1:Th: 038

> T   nee, nee, nou ik hoor het regelmatig hoor dat identiteitskaarten, zo'n kaart
>   die u dan heeft, dat die allang verlengd had moeten worden, maar dat dat nog
>   niet gebeurd is, omdat er zo'n achterstand is
>   *no, no, well I hear it regularly that identity cards, such a card as you have then,*
>   *that it should already have been extended but that that did not happen yet be-*
>   *cause there is such a backlog*

> I   mīgūyand ke az kasān-e dīgarī ham īšān šenīdand ke eqāmatešān bāyad
> tamdīd mīšod, montahā yek moddatī tamdīd našode, montazerand dalīl ān
> ham īn ast ke al'ān yek meqdārī kār-e dādgostarī 'aqab oftāde, čūn sarešān
> kheylī šolūgh ast
> *he says that he from other people also he heard that their residence permit had
> to be extended but for a while has not been extended, they wait, the reason for
> that is that is that at this moment a bit the work of Justice has a backlog, because
> they are very busy*

As was seen in the previous examples, the interpreter adds "he says" at the beginning of his turn, indicating the therapist's space. In this case, however, the perspective changes. The therapist is talking about himself, indicating himself with "I,"
first person. The interpreter, however, changes the perspective and speaks about
"he," thus talking *about* the therapist and turning it into *indirect reported speech*. In
the material examined, this change of perspective is only used in therapists' renditions, when a therapist speaks about himself as an acting person (this in contrast to
the use of "I" in empathic phrases such as "I understand" or "I can imagine").

3.   Direct translation
Turn 1:P: 015

> P   na īnke moškel rā man īyād kardam khob man ham yek meqdārî delšowre
> wa delšowre bāyad dāšte bāšam, šāyad aslan ministerie nakhāhad dobāre yek
> sāl-e dīgar īn kārt rā tamdīd konad
> *not that I caused the problem, now I also a little worried and I have to be wor-
> ried, perhaps in general the Ministry does not want for another year renew this
> card*
>
> I   het is, eh, inderdaad een probleem dat niets met mij te maken heeft, maar in
> ieder geval ben ik bang voor de gevolgen daarvan, want stel dat Justitie dat
> nog een jaar niet verlengt [...]
> *it is, eh, indeed a problem that has nothing to do with me, but in any case I
> am afraid for the effects of it, because, suppose that Justice that again does not
> renew for a year [...]*

In the above example, the interpreter uses the same perspective of person and does
not add an explicit space builder. This example comes from the sessions with the
interpreter who ascribed the "inert vessel" style of assessing interpreted speech to
the therapist. He assumes that the therapist understands that these words come
from the patient and is just *repeating* them in a different language, in keeping with
the officially preferred style, as mentioned above.

4.   Indirect translation
Turn 5:P: 003

> P   barādaram marīz būd. dīdan-e barādaram raftam, taklīfi ziyād dāšt dīdan-i
> az ū ham raftam, pā-ye khodam ham bisyār čī šode būd, hamī qismat bīkhī
> šārīde būd. bisyār ziyād ke hīč namītawānestam begaštam, raftam khāne-ye
> barādaram, moddat-e taqrīban se hafte hamūnjā māndam, ke hamrāham yak
> zare komak kardand ke pā-ye mā hīč namīpūšīdam. faqat esterāhat
> *my brother was ill, I went to visit my brother, he had many complaints, I went to*
> *see him, my own leg also was not well, this part was totally scratched, very much so*
> *that I could not walk, I went to the house of my brother, about three weeks I stayed,*
> *they have helped me a little, I have not used my leg at all, I only rested a bit*
>
> I   ja, twee redenen, ten eerste hij was naar zijn broer gegaan wij eh omdat broer
> ziek was en dat was eh goede steun voor hem als meneer bij was en ten twee
> hij had zelf ook heel veel last van zijn been en hij is naar Amsterdam gegaan
> dan hoefde hij die kunstbeen niet te gebruiken een tijdje, drie weken lang
> *yes, two reasons, firstly he had gone to his brother, we eh because brother was ill*
> *and that was eh good support for him when mister was with him and second he*
> *had himself a lot of trouble with his leg and he is gone to Amsterdam so he did*
> *not have to use that artificial leg for a while, three weeks long*

Here the interpreter does not use a reporting verb. The "yes" can be seen as an implicit space builder. Apart from other changes introduced by the interpreter, the perspective of person is changed from first to third person. The patient speaks for himself in the first person, the interpreter talks *about* the patient turning the utterance into a report of what the patient said.

5.2 Change in perspective in practice: Combinations of the four strategies

In the material, interpreters sometimes use combinations of these four strategies when interpreting a single turn. The following combinations occur regularly.

1.   Multiple representation: the interpreter does not make do with adding "s/he says" at the beginning of a turn, but uses the formulation more often. This varies from using it a second time at the beginning of a new information unit within a turn, or when the primary speaker changes the perspective, to adding it 14 times in a single turn of 70 words in the source language. The "s/he says" formulation may appear right at the beginning of the interpreted turn, but may also be interspersed following a few words of (in)direct translation.

2.   Mixed translation: here the interpreter holds the same perspective as the primary speaker in part of the turn, but then shifts to a different perspective, as in the following example:

Turn 6:P: 013

> P   wa az īn man mītarsam ke khodā na karda dar āyande man az hamīn yak qesmat-e badan falaj našawam
> *and I am afraid that from this part of my body, God forbid, not to get paralyzed*
> I   krijgt heel veel pijn als hij slaapt en hij, zijn angst is misschien is de toekomst word ik invalide
> *gets a lot of pain when he sleeps and he, his fear is perhaps in the future I become an invalid*

"He" and "I" in the interpreter's turn both refer to the same person.

3.   Mixed translation/representation
This combination appears in turns that are longer than a single "sentence." The interpreter starts with a translation form, only to add the "s/he says" formulation later in the turn. Direct and indirect translations both appear in this combination within one turn.

6.   Interpreters' styles of dealing with change in perspective

The three interpreters use the above-identified strategies of perspective change at different frequencies, as shown in Table 2. The form used most frequently by all three interpreters is **direct representation**. The interpreter starts with "he says," after which he provides a direct translation, retaining the same perspective of person as that of the primary speaker. This form, including multiple representation, is nearly always used for renditions of therapists' turns.

In the interview, Interpreter One expressed his explicit strategy of using a reporting verb for therapist renditions and direct translation for patient renditions. This amounts to a "recipient design," in which "the talk by a party in a conversation is constructed or designed in ways which display an orientation and sensitivity to

Table 2. Strategies of change of perspective of person per interpreter and primary speaker, in percentages (figures adapted from Haarhuis 2003)

		Direct representation	Direct translation	Indirect representation	Indirect translation	Other
Interpreter One	Therapist	86	5	5	1	3
	Patient	0	94	0	1.5	4.5
Interpreter Two	Therapist	81	17	0	1	1
	Patient	54	27	0	2	17
Interpreter Three	Therapist	94	2	0	0	4
	Patient	24	38	2	19	17

the particular other(s) who are the (co)participants" (Sacks et al. 1978: 43). Interpreters Two and Three predominantly use a direct representation in their renditions of therapist turns — just like Interpreter One — but use several strategies when rendering patient turns.

The next most frequent form is **direct translation**, which Interpreters One and Three use predominantly for their renditions of patient turns and Interpreter Two uses for both primary speakers. Indirect forms are infrequent: **indirect representation** (which equals indirect reported speech) is used several times, as in "he said he would come." Interpreters One and Two rarely use it at all. Interpreter Three mainly uses **indirect translation** when rendering patient turns. This leads to a narrative style in which he talks about the patient: "he went to see his brother." Interpreters Two and Three use combined strategies most often, while Interpreter One does so only rarely.

According to the translation-machine model of interpreting, the perspective of person should remain unchanged. Following a strict definition, the use of a reporting verb would assign a rendition to the interactive model. At first, the use of a reporting verb also seemed to indicate a change in perspective. However, the findings show a frequent co-occurrence of reporting verb and direct translation. The reporting verb does not represent a change in perspective as such, but is an explicit "space builder." The words of the primary speaker appear as an "embedded space" (Sanders 1994:18), within which the perspective is unchanged as compared to the primary utterance.

Including the use of a reporting verb in the translation-machine model (thus including both the direct representation and the direct translation) means that all three interpreters follow this model in most of their renditions as far as the perspective of person is concerned. Interpreter Three is the only one who quite frequently deviates from it when rendering the turns of the patient.

7.   A specific change of perspective

Most changes in perspective relate to a shift from first person to third, but in the sessions of Patient Two, another change is noticed: the patient addresses the therapist in the third person (talking about "he" and "him"), and this is rendered by Interpreter Two in the second person. This type of change occurs only once in all the renditions of patient turns by Interpreters One and Three.

Patient Two addresses the therapist more often than the other two patients do. This happens mostly in the second session and presumably reflects the fact that the patient is very upset with the therapist for something that was said in an earlier session. After the initial greeting, the patient immediately raises this subject.

Turn 4:P: 004

> P   bale, [eh], haqīq̌ateš man az dast-e āqā kheylī ʿasābānīyam [I: bebakhšīd]
> montahā tebq-e maʾmūl bā ʿasābānīyat raftam bīrūn
> *yes, eh, to be honest I'm very angry with Mister Z [Int says "sorry"] but as usual*
> *I went with my anger outside*
>
> I   hij zegt, eerlijk gezegd, ik ben heel erg boos op de heer Z, maar zoals gebrui-
> kelijk ondanks die boosheid probeer ik toch te glimlachen.
> *he says, to be honest, I'm very angry with Mister Z but as usual despite the anger*
> *I still try to smile*

Here the patient refers to the therapist as "Mister Z," using the third person. The interpreter uses a direct representation, leaving the third person intact. The patient then continues with three long turns, talking continuously about "him," indicating the therapist. These turns are all rendered indirectly, and in some turns a representation form is also used. The change in perspective is from third to second person singular. The patient talks to the interpreter *about* the therapist, but the interpreter translates as if the patient had addressed the therapist directly. The therapist reacts, addressing the patient in the second person, and this is rendered as a direct representation (there is not much choice in rendering second person). In the next six turns, the patient again talks about the therapist in the third person. These turns are rendered again in second person singular.

After these six turns, the therapist has two consecutive turns. Then the patient talks again about the therapist as "Mister Z," and this is rendered as a direct translation. Later, the patient has two more turns about this subject, where he refers to the therapist in the third person singular, rendered respectively in the third person plural and second person singular. Only once does the interpreter use a representation form to translate these turns. The patient distances himself from the therapist by talking about "he" and "him" but the interpreter does not represent this distance in his renditions; he does not copy the distant form of address "he," nor does he use a reporting verb.

It is tempting to ascribe the use of the third person by the patient to his anger. It might be easier to report this anger to the interpreter than to direct it at the therapist himself — as criticism may be more easily uttered without the criticized person present. However, in the previous session and in other parts of this one, the third person is also used. Only once, asking "what do you mean," does he address the therapist directly. As this use of the third person is hardly ever rendered as such, the therapist is not aware of it. He has arranged the seating in such a way that the patient sits opposite him, while the interpreter sits very close and slightly behind the therapist. The reasoning behind the seating is that it allows the interpreter to work as "an instrument" and allows the patient to address the therapist directly instead of turning to the interpreter. What happens is exactly the opposite.

Whether this has to do with the general demeanor of the patient or is induced by the instrumental attitude towards the interaction remains unclear.

Patients One and Three never use the third person to address the therapist. Patient One addresses the therapist only rarely. In the first session, he asks a clarifying question ("do you mean …"), which is not interpreted. The interpreter answers the question himself by repeating the original question asked by the therapist. In the second session, he refers to the therapist twice. Both times he is looking for words and expresses himself hesitantly, saying things like "you know what I mean?" Neither of these is rendered. Patient Three addresses the therapist more often: 13 times in two sessions, and he always uses the second person. He says, for example, "you know that…" or "as I told you before…." These phrases are generally not rendered, but when they are, the rendition, perhaps inevitably, remains in the second person. It is also tempting to ascribe the use of the third person to address the therapist to the cultural background of the patient, but the other two patients, who have the same cultural background, do not use this form of address. Although the interpreter does not present it as a conscious decision, he has chosen to change the perspective, and in this case it leads to a different presentation of the patient–therapist relationship than when originally worded.

8.   Multiple representation

The use of a representation form, i.e. the addition of a reporting verb, is widespread in the data collected. Interpreters frequently use a representation form not just once at the beginning of a rendition as an explicit space builder — meaning "what follows belongs to the base space of the preceding primary speaker" — but also in the course of the rendition. The use of this perspective varies among interpreters, but is more widespread in renditions of therapists' turns, as can be seen in Table 3.

Table 3. The use of reporting verbs by the three interpreters

Represent	Renditions of therapist turns			Renditions of patient turns		
	Total*	Single	Multiple	Total	Single	Multiple
Interpreter One	114 /128 89%	79	35	0 /139 0%	0	0
Interpreter Two	114 /170 67%	110	4	64 /109 59%	56	8
Interpreter Three	73 / 102 70%	31	42	60 /184 33%	48	12

* Total = total number of renditions in which one or more reporting verbs has been used/total number of renditions in the two sessions
Single – multiple = number of turns in which one or more than one reporting verb has been used

Although it seems unlikely that the use of more than one reporting verb in a rendition is completely random, the analysis has not revealed a set pattern or a single explanation. The use of multiple representation by each interpreter is discussed below.

8.1 Interpreter One

Interpreter One's use of representation, and thus of multiple representation, is limited to his renditions of therapist's turns, and bears some relationship to the length of the turn. The average total turn length is 21 words, whereas the average length of turns in which multiple representation is used is 35. Still, length of turn is not the only determinant of multiple representation nor is the number of "s/he says" formulations directly related to the length of the turn. There are 11-word turns that are assigned two reporting verbs, and there is also a 66-word turn with two reporting verbs. The next example shows one such short turn:

Turn 2:Th:027

> T   zijn vrouw, in ieder geval, maar u bedoelt misschien iets anders?
> *his wife, in any case, but you mean maybe something else?*
> I   mīgūyand ke khānomešān ke hastand, montahā mīgūyand manzūretān az kasī šāyad kashā-ye dīgarī bāšand
> *he says that his wife is there though, but he says your intention with somebody else maybe other people is*

The therapist reacts to the patient who has just said that his father had nobody around to help him. The therapist's utterance is rendered more elaborately: The "some<u>thing</u>" is changed into a "some<u>body</u>" and "other people," thus focusing the question more on "person." The use of two reporting verbs may reflect the interpreter's difficulty in rendering the turn, and his need to gain time in order to think.

The following example also indicates that difficulty is a factor influencing multiple representation. It concerns a longer turn, of 32 words, that is rendered with three reporting verbs. Before the interpreter begins his rendition, he utters something inaudible, which the therapist understands as a request for clarification. The therapist repeats a word and provides a substitute.

Turn 2:Th: 116

> T   en daardoor kon u eigenlijk het verdriet, wat u had na de gevangenis, kon u eigenlijk niet met haar delen, wat er eigenlijk overbleef, dat waren die rancuneuze, gevoelens die u had

> *and in that way you could in fact not share the sadness, that you had after the*
> *prison, you could in fact not share it with her, what stayed in fact, that were*
> *those rancorous feelings that you had*

I   [inaudible]

T   die rancuneuze, die wraakgevoelens die u had
> *those rancorous, those revenge-feelings that you had*

I   mīgūyand ke šomā pas čūn ān masa'el rā nemīkhāstīd be khānometān qablan
     begū'īd wa mīkhāstīd wāse-ye khodetān negah dârīd, mīgūyand dar wāqe'
     nemītawānestīd ān nārāhatī rā taqsīm bekonîd bā khânometān wa mīgūyand
     be hamān dalīl ham dar wāqe' ān ehsās-e enteqāmgīrī ham dar šomā būd
> *he says that you so because those things you did not want to tell earlier to your*
> *wife and because you wanted to keep everything for yourself, he says in fact you*
> *could not share that sadness with your wife and he says for the same reason also*
> *in fact the revenge-feeling was in you*

A similar case is found in a therapist's 58-word turn which receives six "s/he says"
formulations in the rendition. The fact that this interpreter never uses a reporting
verb when rendering a patient's turns shows, however, that the relationship with
properties of the turn is only relative. The turns of the patient are on average much
longer than those of the therapist (33 versus 20 words), which would make their
rendition more difficult. In general, translating into the mother tongue is supposed to be easier and more natural than working in the other direction ("Nairobi
Declaration", in Shuttleworth 1997: 111; Lonsdale 2001). This would imply that the
therapist's turns are easier for this interpreter to translate than the patient's. It also
supports the expectation that the interpreter will use more reporting verbs in the
patient's renditions. If "difficulty" and "length of the turn" were decisive factors,
he would use a reporting verb more often when rendering the patient's turns than
when rendering the therapist's. In his use of reporting verbs, the interpreter shows
that recipient design, i.e. adapting one's conversational behavior to that of the person addressed, is a decisive factor. He always uses a reporting verb when interpreting the therapist and never when interpreting the patient, even when the patient's
turns are long and have to be rendered in the interpreter's second language. It may
also be an indication that the interpreter finds the patients' words easier to understand than the therapist's.

8.2 Interpreter Two

Interpreter Two uses a reporting verb in his renditions of both the therapist and
the patient. Only rarely does he use multiple reporting verbs: in 4 therapist and 8
patient turns. In the case of the patient, this relates six times to a long turn (longer
than 50 words) and in one case, to a false start. For the therapist, it concerns a false
start once. The other cases follow the format of the following example:

Turn 4:Th: 011

> T even voor de duidelijkheid [.] hetgene wat u aangaf wat zo, wat uw zoon wil zeggen van dat hij mag gillen en schreeuwen tegen u, ik kan me niet herinneren dat ik dat zo met hem besproken heb, maar het lijkt me verstandig dat we daar met zijn drieën daar een gesprek over hebben.
>
> *just for the sake of clarity [.] that what you indicated what so, what your son wants to say of that he may scream and yell to you, I cannot remember that I discussed it with him in that way, but it seems reasonable to me that we have a talk about that with the three of us*
>
> I mīgūyand, hālā barā-ye wāzehīyat, mīgūyand, masāʾelî ke man be pesaretān gofte bāšam ke ejāze dārad dād bezanad saretān, man aslan yādam memīyāyad ke ham čenīn čīzī gofte bāšam, fekr mīkonam ʿāqelāne bāšad ke mā seh nafarī dar īn mowzūʾ sohbat konīm
>
> *he says, now for the clarity, he says what I would have said to your son that he permission to scream to you, I do not remember at all that I would have said something like that, I think that it would be reasonable when we, three persons, talk about this subject*

In all these turns the therapist starts with an introduction. The interpreter starts with a reporting verb and repeats it before the remainder of the turn, though not in all cases. In the case of the patient, the interpreter uses multiple reporting verbs in some long turns, but most often he does not.

8.3 Interpreter Three

Interpreter Three not only uses a reporting verb in a large number of turns, but also uses the "s/he says" formulation very often within a single rendition. Like interpreters One and Two, he uses a reporting verb more frequently in therapist turns — in 70 % versus in 33 % of the cases of the patient. In his renditions of the patient, use of multiple representation is limited to two or three reporting verbs. In therapist turns, six or seven reporting verbs in the rendition of a single turn are not uncommon. In one (extreme) case "he says" is used 14 times in a single 72-word turn.

When asked, the interpreter does not offer any explanation for his frequent use of "he says" and does not seem particularly aware of it. As previously noted, "s/he says" at the beginning of a rendition serves as an explicit space builder, indicating that what follows stems from the base space of the immediately preceding speaker. However, when it is inserted every few words, "s/he says" probably no longer serves this purpose, as the listener does not need frequent reminders of the mental space that is being elucidated. I have the impression — and this is also based on my analysis of the quality of the renditions, not presented in the present paper — that the use of multiple representations is linked to the difficulties the interpreter encounters in translating the therapist turns, and that "s/he says" may serve primarily to provide a thinking pause.

8.4 Concluding multiple representations

All three interpreters use multiple representations mostly when rendering therapist turns, even though these turns are shorter than those of the patient, and even though all three interpreters have Dutch as their second language. Besides the strong recipient design of Interpreter One (described above), the findings seem to indicate that the interventions of the therapist are more difficult for the interpreters to understand than the narratives of the patients.

9. Conclusions

Although all three interpreters use direct translations in a number of cases, thus showing that the basic idea of "repeating the primary turns" is an accepted concept, deviations from this ideal of direct translation in this material are widespread, despite the emphasis placed upon it by the international professional community. Interpreters very often do not *repeat* what the primary speakers said in a different language, as they are expected to do; rather, in many cases they *report* what the primary speakers said in a different language.

All three interpreters have their own style of indicating that they are not the authors of the words they speak. Their strategy depends on such factors as turn length and/or structure, difficulty, and ideas about the recipient's understanding.

Interpreter One follows the strictest strategy: a direct representation in renditions of the therapist turns, a direct translation in the renditions of the patient's — with few exceptions. He has adopted this recipient-design strategy to fit the listener. Interpreter Two does not follow a strict recipient design, but uses direct representations and direct translations for both primary speakers. Interpreter Three uses indirect translations quite frequently for the patient, along with direct translations and direct representations. For his renditions of therapist turns, he makes frequent recourse to representation forms, and very frequently uses multiple reporting verbs.

Most often the deviations from the "direct rule" thus take the form of "direct reported speech," in which the interpreter begins with a reporting verb and then provides a direct translation of the preceding primary turn. The reporting verb serves as an "explicit space builder," indicating that the embedded space belongs to the "base space" of the preceding primary speaker. The use of a reporting verb (and of indirect translation) is generally seen as a way for interpreters to distance themselves from the words they render. However, when the use of reporting verbs is so widespread, as was the case in all six sessions examined, it loses its discriminating power and does not serve as a method of creating distance from *specific* utterances of the primary speakers. As a direct representation leaves the embedded space intact, it can be concluded that the mere addition of a reporting verb does not detract from the impartial position of the interpreter. It merely emphasizes that the interpreter is part of the dialogue and at the same time defines his position as "reporter."

In conclusion, the findings do not reveal any reason not to include the use of a reporting verb at the beginning of a rendition in the definition of "good interpreting practice." Nor does an occasional change from first to third person appear to compromise the interpretation. Opponents of changes in perspective of person and the addition of reporting verbs mention its alienating effect and its distancing of the primary speakers. When the analysis of the findings described here was presented at the 4th Critical Link Conference in Stockholm (May 2004), it met with much resistance. Participants opposed my lenient attitude towards the use of a reporting verb and to changes from the first to third person. The opponents' argument rested primarily on the great importance, in psychotherapy, of direct contact between therapist and patient. While the importance of this contact is undeniable, is it not a myth that in interpreter-mediated talk the primary speakers are communicating directly? These changes are a reflection of the nature of the dialogue, which is after all three-party talk, though with a specific flavour. In fact, a complete rejection of the idea of a change in perspective of person would indicate a belief in the translation-machine model. This may lead to the denial of the three-party character of the interaction that does take place and may eventually compromise the quality of the interaction.

The effect of frequent indirect translation and multiple use of reporting verbs — the strategy employed most frequently by Interpreter Three — could not be ascertained on the basis of these findings. It appears, however, that when "s/he says" is used more often than once within a single turn, it loses its function as a space builder and may function as a "thinking pause." In the sessions of Group 3, the therapist often hears the patient's words through the interpreter in narrative form; the interpreter speaks in the third person about "what is the matter with the patient," and the patient hears the therapist's words presented hesitantly and disjointedly, interspersed with many "s/he says" formulations.

The analysis of the videotaped sessions (Bot, 2005) shows that the sessions of Group Three have more information loss and unresolved misunderstandings between therapist and patient than those of the other two groups. The therapist in these sessions delegates the organization of the sessions largely to the interpreter, and does not interfere when patient talk overlaps with interpreter talk or when the patient continues speaking while the interpreter tries to take the turn. Interpreter Three's use of multiple reporting verbs and of indirect translation seems to be related to the way the participants in this group organize the sessions.

These sessions also show a large percentage of divergent renditions. Together, this gives the interpreter a pivotal role in the dialogue: he not only organizes the structure of the session but also co-defines the content of the interaction. This emphasizes the reported-speech and the constructed-dialogue character of the renditions; the voice of the interpreter looms large. Although I have seen that this is the case to some extent in all six sessions, and although I think that it is inevitable that the interpreter influences the session, I think it is worthwhile to try to limit this influence. This includes limiting changes in the perspective of person. In this article I have isolated one aspect of the dialogue. It is clear that the influence of this aspect on the proceeding of the session can only be assessed in relation to others and in relation to characteristics of the dialogue as a whole.

Notes

1. *"Directe vertaling"* literally means "direct translation." I have learned that in English *direct translation* means a translation from the foreign language into the mother tongue or into a language in which he or she has a mastery equal to that of the mother tongue (Lonsdale 2001: 64). In Dutch interpreting circles, the term is used as described in this article.

2. The Persian and Dari in all examples have been transliterated from the Persian script following the English convention. Transcripts, transliterations and translations into Dutch were made and checked by lecturers of the Departments of Foreign Languages of the Universities of Utrecht and Leiden, both in the Netherlands. The English translations of the Dutch utterances and of the Dutch translations of the Persian and Dari were made by the author. If the grammatical structure of the original was faulty, the English translation will be faulty as well.

3. Turn 4: T: 007 means this turn stems from the fourth recorded session, is a therapist turn and is the seventh turn in the session.

References

Bot, H. (2005). *Dialogue interpreting in mental health*. Amsterdam/New York: Rodopi [Utrecht Series in Language and Communication no. 19].
Bot, H. & Wadensjö, C. (2004). The presence of a third party: A dialogical view on interpreter-assisted treatment. In B. Drosdek & J. Wilson (Eds.), *Broken spirits: The treatment of trau-*

matized asylum seekers, refugees, war and torture victims. New York: Brunner-Routledge, 355–378.

Fauconnier, G. (1985). *Mental spaces: Aspects of meaning construction in natural language.* Cambridge: Cambridge University Press.

Haarhuis, J. (2003). *Perspectiefgebruik van tolken tijdens psychotherapie.* Unpublished MA thesis, Faculty of Arts, University of Utrecht.

Lonsdale, A. B. (2001). Direction of translation (directionality). In M. Baker (Ed.), *Routledge encyclopedia of translation studies.* London/New York: Routledge, 63–67.

Pöchhacker, F. (2004). *Introducing interpreting studies.* London/New York: Routledge.

Roy, C. B. (2000). *Interpreting as a discourse process.* New York/Oxford: Oxford University Press.

Sacks, H. E., Schegloff. E. & Jefferson, G. (1978). A simplest systematics for the organisation of turn-taking for conversation. In J. N. Schenkein (Ed.), *Studies in the organisation of conversational interaction.* New York: Academic Press, 7–55.

Sanders, J. M. (1994). *Perspective in narrative discourse.* PhD dissertation, Katholieke Universiteit Brabant, Tilburg.

Shuttleworth, M. (Ed.) (1997). *Dictionary of translation studies,* Manchester: St. Jerome.

Streeck, J. & Hartge, U. (1992). Previews: Gestures at the transition place. In P. Auer & A. di Luzio (Eds.), *The contextualisation of language.* Amsterdam: John Benjamins, 135–158.

Tannen, D. (1989). *Talking voices, repetition, dialogue and imagery in conversational discourse.* Cambridge: Cambridge University Press.

Wadensjö, C. (1998). *Interpreting as interaction.* London/New York: Longman.

Wallmach, K. (2002). "Seizing the surge of language by its soft bare skull": Simultaneous interpreting, the Truth Commission and Country of My Skull. *Current Writing* (Special issue on Translation and Power) 14 (2), 64–82.

Examining the "voice of interpreting" in speech pathology

Raffaela Merlini and Roberta Favaron[1]
University of Macerata and University of Trieste / ISMETT, Palermo

This paper investigates professional interpreting practice in the setting of speech pathology through a multifaceted analysis of the transcripts of three recorded sessions involving first-generation Italian-speaking immigrants to Australia and English-speaking healthcare professionals working in Melbourne. Applying Mishler's notion of "voice" to the context of interpreter-mediated communication and focusing on a selection of linguistic features — ranging from turn-taking and topic development to the interpreter's choice of footing, departures from the primary speakers' utterances, and use of prosodic resources — the discussion identifies the voice that interpreters, as third participants in the interaction, choose to adopt between the "voice of medicine" and the "voice of the lifeworld". The study is of a qualitative nature, although a general indication of the frequency of certain features is supplied, and interpreting conduct is described rather than prescribed. The reporting and interpretation of findings are, however, informed by and reflect issues of value revolving around the concept of "humane medical care".

1. The study

This study is an attempt to gain insight into how professional interpreters perform their task in a well-defined medical setting. When compared to other institutional contexts, doctor-patient encounters are found to offer a more heterogeneous scenario, in that their "shape, form, trajectory, content or character", in the words of Schegloff (1992: 111), are more open to "local" negotiation between the participants. As will be discussed below, this process may result in alternative discourse models, depending on each participant's choice of his/her own "voice", which in the case of the healthcare professional may be more or less dominant, and more or less detached or "disaffiliative" (Drew & Heritage 1992: 24). The interesting question, from our perspective, is what voice the interpreter will choose to adopt in the ongoing interaction. Before answering this question, however, a brief outline will be drawn of the relevant healthcare setting, namely speech pathology, and of the data used for the analysis.

1.1 The setting

The branch of medical science which falls under the heading of "speech therapy" or "speech pathology" is concerned both with the general physiological and pathological aspects of the speech organs, and with the study and correction of speech defects (Critchley 1978: 1008), which may affect children or may occur at a later stage in life — e.g. following apoplexy and similar traumas. Speech defects are defined as impairments in the ability to (1) receive and/or process, (2) represent, and/or (3) transmit and use symbol systems (Jackson 1988: 257). The job responsibilities of speech pathologists thus range from the identification and assessment of a medical condition to the implementation of appropriate intervention programs, including the organisation of encounters with patients and their relatives.

When speech pathology sessions involve people speaking mutually incomprehensible languages, and an interpreter is called upon to facilitate their interaction, the picture becomes a complex one, for the very reason that language is not only the means, but also the object of communication. When no standard tests are available in the patient's primary language, the speech assessment is traditionally performed through "interest finders", which, depending on the client's age, might range from informal conversation to descriptions of personal experiences. Whilst topics are as close as possible to the patient's everyday life, the linguistic features of the questioning strategy are non-casual, as the aim is to elicit specific language samples, which may be words, phrases or longer sentences (Langdon 2002: 63). To this end, speech pathologists may decide to use either simple yes-or-no questions or open-ended questions, such as "tell me about..." or "how do you...?", which require full sentences to provide a complete answer. Alternatively, patients may be asked to produce narrative samples by retelling stories and movies, or by formulating tales from comic strips and wordless books (Langdon & Cheng 2002: 86–87).

Given the nature of the assessment process, the linguistic skills needed to interpret in this field include not only general requirements such as familiarity with both cultures and with nonverbal communication, and knowledge of professional terminology, but also the ability to reproduce the language of people with speech disorders (see Langdon 2002; Langdon & Cheng 2002). Significantly, while stressing the importance of verbatim translation of the patients' utterances during assessment sessions ("do not edit what is said, and do not change sounds"), Langdon (2002: 7) also urges interpreters to explain to speech pathologists what is said versus what should have been said, thereby helping them recognise the extent and causes of the language impairment and provide appropriate feedback. Gentile et al. (1996: 125–135) further clarify that the interpreter's metalinguistic descriptions may refer to syntax, phonology and semantics.

1.2 The data

The data for this article come from three speech pathology sessions recorded at two healthcare facilities in Melbourne, Australia in 2001, and involve Italian-speaking first-generation immigrants, English-speaking healthcare professionals and in-house NAATI-accredited[2] interpreters. The three sessions, which are part of a wider corpus of 32 interpreted encounters presented elsewhere,[3] are schematically described in Table 1.[4]

Table 1. Summary information about the transcripts

	Transcript 1 (T. 1)	Transcript 2 (T. 2)	Transcript 3 (T. 3)
Place	Extended Care Centre, Melbourne	Extended Care Centre, Melbourne	General Hospital, Melbourne
Date	21 March 2001	12 July 2001	13 July 2001
Duration	10' 30"	25' 25"	18' 05"
Partici-pants	– female speech pathol-ogist, aged 25 (*Sheila*); – male in-patient, aged 80–90, affected by speech disorder, caused by apoplexy (*Patrizio*); – female in-house inter-preter, aged 43 (*Ines*).	– female speech pathol-ogist, aged 25 (*Sheila*); – male in-patient, aged 80, affected by speech disor-der, caused by apoplexy (*Pino*); – female in-house inter-preter, aged 43 (*Ines*).	– female speech pathol-ogist, aged 30 (*Sara*); – male in-patient, aged 80, affected by speech disor-der, caused by apoplexy (*Pietro*); – female in-house inter-preter, aged 50 (*Ippolita*); – patient's wife.
Purpose	assessment of swallowing difficulties and explanation of future medical checks	therapy session	therapy session

Some observations must be made concerning the nature of the encounters. Since their purpose is either a routine check on an in-patient's condition, followed by an explanation of future diagnostic tests, as in T.1, or therapy with long-term patients, as in T.2 and T.3, all three sessions deviate substantially from the samples used in most studies of monolingual doctor-patient interaction, which focus almost exclusively on first meetings where the aim is history-taking and diagnosis of a current complaint. The specificity of the interactional contexts, where the medical practitioners are relating to patients they know, will have to be taken into account in the following analysis. Secondly, as we move from T.1 to T.3, the conditions affecting the three patients become progressively more severe, to the extent that, if Patrizio is fully able to converse, Pino utters simple sentences in response to the speech pathologist's questions, whereas Pietro only whispers single words, which are at times almost inaudible.

The transcription conventions applied in this paper are largely based upon the model first developed by Gail Jefferson (see Atkinson & Heritage 1984: ix–xvi). However, as each notation system is the reflection of specific research goals, some symbols have been left out as irrelevant (e.g. those indicating aspirations, inhalations and gutturalness), others have been modified (e.g. signs representing pauses) and a few added (e.g. fillers, which have also been assigned fixed meanings following Eggins & Slade 1997: 3). (For the full transcription key, see the Appendix). Recordings were transcribed jointly by the present authors, who returned regularly to the audiotapes to test and evaluate their analyses and interpretations.

2. The theoretical framework

The availability of recorded sessions spawned the idea of a qualitative study[5] based mainly, though not entirely, on the investigation concerns of conversation analysis (hereafter CA). As a prelude to using some of the conceptual tools of this well-established research tradition, we will recall here the emphasis it places on the sequential nature of talk — on its being made up of "sequences" of activity emerging dynamically from the interplay between smaller units ("turns-within-sequences"; Drew & Heritage 1992: 18), also referred to as the "contiguity principle" (Fele 1999: 38–39). Through detailed and intensive analysis of naturally occurring conversation — an empirical perspective which has been the hallmark of CA since its appearance in the 1970s — researchers have come to the conclusion that the interpretation of an utterance as an *action* does not depend on some elusive, intrinsic quality, but on preceding and successive turns in the conversation. In other words, each turn has a retrospective effect, in that it sheds light on what was previously said, as well as a prospective function, in that it projects the expectation that an appropriate response will be provided so that a given sequence may be continued or completed.

With reference to institutional talk, more specifically to medical encounters, the interest in how turns are taken and topics shifted by physicians and patients directed us to two seminal studies: Mishler (1984) and Fairclough (1992). Whilst the contribution of the latter to the present paper will become evident in the next section, Mishler's approach was also a source of inspiration at a more general level.

The author presented us with the theoretical notion of "voice", which was found to offer a flexible interpretative framework as well as a ready-made metaphorical association to our field of study, speech pathology.

Without following Mishler's line of theorising through to his adoption of Habermas' (1970)[6] socio-political perspective, we have borrowed his basic distinction between two analytic categories, the "voice of the lifeworld" and the "voice of medicine" (henceforth VoL and VoM). Starting from an initial definition of "voice" as an ensemble of "relationships between talk and speakers' underlying frameworks of meaning" (1984: 14), Mishler uses the former label to refer to the expression of and attention to concerns stemming from events and problems of everyday life. In contrast, VoM designates an abstract, affectively neutral and functionally specific[7] interpretation of facts, as well as compliance with a "normative order", whereby the professional controls both content and organization of the interaction.[8] It should be noted that the two voices do not necessarily coincide with that of the patient and of the healthcare practitioner, respectively. Often it will be the physician who, being equally competent in both codes, decides to speak in either the VoM or the VoL, displaying a lower vs. higher degree of attentiveness to the patient's understanding of reality and communicative needs.

Whereas in a monolingual encounter, the "burden" of translating between the two voices generally falls on the physician, in cross-lingual and intercultural communication, dynamics become more complex with the appearance of a third voice, which will be referred to here as the "voice of interpreting" (VoI). The picture would be relatively unproblematic if the VoI were seen to confine itself to echoing the other two through a mechanical translation pattern, whereby each utterance in the source language is transformed into an equivalent utterance in the target language. But what if this were not the case and the VoI were found to express a separate identity, not only by conveying the needs of its own operational mode, but by altering a primary speaker's selection of either the VoL or the VoM? In the first instance, we could even contemplate the case of the interpreter's clients using the VoI to express their acknowledgment of the difficulties, limitations and requirements of the interpreting process; in the second instance, the reinforcement, at the interpreting stage, of either the VoM or the VoL and, more radically, the conversion of one voice into another would signify an expansion of the VoI's scope. This would come to coincide with the voice of a third participant making independent choices between the alternatives available at any one point in the interaction, on the basis of his/her own analysis of the participants' communicative goals and needs.

In order to investigate the ways in which the three voices interact with one another, our analysis of the recorded sessions will include some linguistic features which are absent in Mishler's study, and exclude others to which he resorts. Hence, although the same attention will be paid to participants' behaviours in interactional management, the interpreter's conversational stances in terms of footing, her[9] additions to the original speakers' utterances and use of prosodic resources will equally be examined.

3.   The voice of interpreting: Analysis and exemplification

For the sake of a clearer exposition, the analysis will proceed through progressive steps along a pathway leading from sequences to single utterances and parts of them, to words and, finally, to prosodic features. It should, however, be pointed out that the levels of enquiry are not impermeable categories and will often show ample areas of overlap — a prime example of this is the case of autonomous interventions by the interpreter, which can be described from three different perspectives, turn-taking, footing and additions. Although these aspects will first be treated separately, in the conclusions an attempt will be made to present some of their combined effects. Owing to constraints of length, only one example will be offered for most of the points raised in the following paragraphs.

3.1 Turn-taking and topic control

Though opting for an alternative interpretative framework, in his discussion of "standard"[10] vs. "alternative" medical interviews, Fairclough (1992) makes use of CA tools to construct his argumentation — i.e. that the ongoing shift in medical practice seems to be away from a model of interaction where the professionals overtly exercise their authority, towards a non-directive, informal approach, which underlines treating the patient as a person and not as a case, giving him or her space to talk and empathising with his or her account; in other words, a shift from the dominance of the VoM towards the VoL.

First among CA concepts is that of *adjacency pair* — a more general structural type than Sinclair and Coulthard's (1975) "exchanges" — which was first developed by Schegloff and Sacks (1973). Of all the adjacency pairs which have been studied in subsequent CA literature, the question-answer pattern has been recurrently identified as the predominant discursive format in many institutional settings. Doctor-patient interviews, in particular, have been shown to proceed through a recursive chain of interlinked pairings, giving rise to characteristic three-part sequences of question-response-acknowledgment (Mishler 1984; Silverman 1987; Frankel 1990). Moving from diagnostic interviews to the context of speech therapy, this basic sequence takes the slightly modified form of speech pathologist's question — patient's response — speech pathologist's assessment.

The obvious effect of a framework of this kind is that the doctor controls the **turn-taking** system, i.e. the way talking turns are distributed between participants. In their seminal study on turn-taking, Sacks, Schegloff and Jefferson (1974) propose a simple but powerful system consisting of two components: turn-constructional units and an ordered set of turn-allocation rules. The current speaker in an interaction constructs his/her turn with grammatical units, such as sentences, clauses, phrases or even single words, and other participants are able to determine the type of unit and predict its point of completion, i.e. the point — called "transition-relevance place" or TRP — where the floor is again potentially available.[11] At these points, the following rules apply: (1) the current speaker may select the next speaker, for instance by addressing him/her; (2) if this does not happen, the next speaker may self-select by taking the floor; (3) if this does not happen, the current speaker may continue. Whilst in ordinary conversation these options are equally available to all participants, institutional interaction often exhibits an asymmetrical distribution of talking rights and obligations between "powerful" (P) and "non-powerful" (N-P) participants, whereby, as Fairclough observes (1992: 153):

> (i)   P may select N-P, but not vice-versa; (ii) P may self-select, but N-P may not; […] (iii) P's turn may be extended across any number of points of possible completion.

With reference to medical encounters, what this means in practice is that the patient usually takes the floor when the doctor offers it by asking him a question. The doctor, in contrast, is not given the floor, but takes it when the patient has finished answering the question, or when she decides that the patient's response has become "irrelevant" to a strictly medical assessment of his problem. In the latter case, *overlaps* may be used by the doctor as a device to cut short the patient's turn. If, on the other hand, no response is given by the patient and the question is followed by a *pause*, the doctor may take the floor again to urge the patient to supply an answer. A corollary of this organisation relates to **topic control**. It is the doctor who introduces new topics through her questions, "polices the agenda" (Fairclough 1992: 155) by assessing, either explicitly or implicitly, the patient's answer, changes topic by interrupting the patient, or stays on topic by repeating the same question to counter the patient's silence.

In a less asymmetrical interactional format, as is displayed in the "alternative" medical interview studied by Fairclough (1992: 144–149), turn-taking is shown to be more collaboratively managed and topic development more extensively negotiated by the two participants. However, this is made possible only by the doctor's willingness to make the floor available to the patient. This sensitivity does not mean that she is surrendering interactional control, as the author acutely observes (1992:146):

> Notice that the initiative for yielding a measure of control to the patient in medical interviews of this sort invariably comes from the doctor, which suggests that doctors do still exercise control at some level, even if in the paradoxical form of ceding control.

If in a monolingual context "yielding a measure of control" to the patient can be a matter of personal choice between a more or less empathic, more or less formal, more or less directive interactional model, in linguistically mediated encounters professionals may have little or no alternative to ceding some of their control tools to the interpreter. The following paragraphs will illustrate the ways in which the interpreters, in particular in sessions 2 and 3, are actively involved in managing the exchange of turns as well as information between the primary interlocutors. The idea of organising examples into three sections — smooth transitions, pauses, and overlaps — is taken from Roy's (1996) inspiring article on turn-taking at an interpreted event involving American Sign Language.

Smooth transitions

The fact that interpreter-mediated encounters entail a specific turn-taking order to account for the interpreter's translation[12] may seem an obvious enough statement. What is not so obvious, however, is that the absence or delay of the interpreter's turn would be a noticeable occurrence or, as the case may be, a noticeable non-occurrence. This suggests that in an interpreted interaction, the above-mentioned concept of adjacency pair needs revisiting to account for a doubling up of actions which are expected to occur as a logical continuation of the first part of the pair. In other words, the utterance of a primary speaker "sequentially implicates" not only the utterance of the other primary speaker, but, prior to this, the translating act of the interpreter. We would therefore submit that a more appropriate way to designate this double implicature might be *adjacency trio*.[13]

In our field of study, one would expect the *unmarked* forms of this pattern to be:

1. SP's question — I's translation — P's answer
2. P's answer — I's translation — SP's assessment / SP's next question
(3. SP's assessment — I's translation — SP's next question)

where SP stands for speech pathologist, I for interpreter and P for patient. The variant in point 2 refers to the case in which the patient's response is implicitly acknowledged as correct by the therapist's simply proceeding to a new question.

Sequence 3 is therefore marked as optional. The following excerpt illustrates a standard sequence of turns smoothly following upon one another, with no disruptions, such as pauses or overlaps:

[1]   T. 2 (189–195)[14]
189 SP: what would you need if you wanted to build some shelves
190 I: ecco che cosa occo:rre (.) se lei vole:sse (.) fare (.) una:: una libreria (.)
           now what would you need if you wanted to make a bookcase
191   °che cosa le occorre (.) per farla°
           what would you need to make it
192 P: umm (del) legno
           some wood
193 I: wood
194 SP: mhm that's right
195 I: sì °giusto°
           yes right

From the point of view of the present study, however, a more interesting feature is the presence of *marked* patterns, where the progression of actions described above is in some way altered. In the following excerpt, for instance, the interpreter does not translate the patient's first answer. Instead, she asks him whether he really has no trees in his garden. The resulting pattern is thus: P's answer — I's question.[15]

[2]   T. 2 (92–96)
92   SP: °mhm° (.) what type of trees and flowers do you have in the garden
93   I: che:: quali alberi che tipo di a::lberi quali fio::ri↑ ha ⌐in giardino ⌐
           which trees what kinds of trees which flowers do you have |*in your garden*|
94   P: └alberi no ┘ alberi no
                                                                          no trees   *no trees*

95   I: **non ce l'ha alberi↑**
           don't you have any trees
96   P: yeah

Soon after, she explicitly acknowledges Pino's answer as correct through the agreement token "mhm", translates for the SP, and then asks Pino what kind of trees they are. The sequence can be represented as: P's answer — I's assessment — I's translation — I's next question.

[3]   T. 2 (95–98)
95   I: **non ce l'ha alberi↑**
           don't you have any trees
96   P: yeah
97   I: **mhm uh I have trees mhm che tipo (.) sono (.) li conosce↑**
                                 what type are they do you know them
98   P: come i fichi↑
           such as figs

Again a few lines later, Ines, after translating for Sheila, gives an implicit assessment of Pino's answer by asking him to provide further examples of the trees which grow

in his garden. The pattern is slightly modified into: P's answer — I's translation
— I's next question.

```
[4]   T. 2 (98–101)
 98   P:    come i fichi↑
            such as figs
 99   I:    fi – fichi↑
            figs
100   P:    yeah=
101   I:    =uh fig fig tree ((addressing the patient)) poi↑ altri↑
                                                        then others
```

Through her interactional conduct, Ines thus exhibits the characteristic behaviour
of a powerful participant, according to Fairclough's rules, in that she self-selects as
next speaker, extends her turns across points of completion and re-allocates the
floor to the patient. Her bypassing the SP's assessment and controlling of topic development could also be viewed as the adoption by the VoI of the typical contours
of the VoM.

Also worthy of note are sequences containing the SP's assessment. Contrary to
the findings of several studies on dialogue interpreting, which identify the extensive omission of feedback parts of utterances by interpreters as one of the trouble
sources of this kind of interaction (see for instance Englund Dimitrova 1997: 160,
and Wadensjö 1998: 236), the analysis of our transcripts has revealed a general
tendency towards conveying them. Ines, for instance, is frequently seen to either
translate Sheila's favourable assessment of the patient's response, as in [1] line 195,
or in the case of non-lexical discourse markers, such as "mhm", repeat it, as shown
in the following example:

```
[5]   T. 2 (303–309)
303   SP:   tell me (.) two things you could buy at a liquor shop
304   I:    ecco un negozio da una enoteca dove si vendono °insomma° dei liquori (.) che
            now in a shop in a wine shop where they sell liquors what
305         cosa potrebbe (.) comprare
            could you buy
306   P:    (oh il) vino
            wine
307   I:    the wine
308   SP:   mhm=
309   I:    =mhm
```

Whilst it is true that in therapy sessions feedback does not have a mere phatic function,[16] but generally carries semantic content, the systematic and often exuber-
ant acknowledgment of the patients' correct answers by both speech pathologists
speaks of an empathic communication model, in which the emotional distancing
of the VoM is supplanted by the affective involvement of the VoL. In this light, the
interpreter's decision to reiterate the therapists' positive feedback, although the

English expressions are perfectly comprehensible to the patients, is, in our view, more than just a professional reflex towards scrupulous word-for-word translation. This reading is supported by the observation of Ippolita's behaviour in T.3. As illustrated in the following excerpt, she starts off by translating only questions and answers and leaving out Sara's feedback expressions:

[6]   T. 3   (34–44)
```
34   SP:   is your name Pietro
35   I:    si chiama Pietro
           is your name Pietro
36         ((the patient nods))
37   SP:   very good (.) is your name umm D'Aquino
38   I:    si ch — il nome è D'Aquino↑
           is your name D'Aquino
39         ((the patient nods))
40   SP:   okay is your name Marcuccio
41   I:    il suo nome è Marcuccio↑
           is your name Marcuccio
42         ((the patient shakes his head))
43   SP:   °okay° ((soft chuckle)) very good Pi:::etro are you a man
44   I:    lei è un uomo Pietro↑
           are you a man Pietro
```

Then, as the session unfolds, she shifts to a more involved model, in the wake of Sara's example:

[7]   T. 3   (288–299)
```
288   SP:   show me the keys
289   I:    e le chia:vi↑
            and the keys
290         ((the patient points to the keys))
291   SP:   that's right
292   I:    bene:
            good
293   SP:   a:nd show me: the watch
294   I:    e l'orologio
            and the watch
295         ((the patient points to the watch))
296   SP:   very good ⌈very good
297   I:              ⌊bravo
                       well done
298   SP:   °without any problems°
299   I:    bravo senza problemi
            well done without any problems

            (325–327)
325   I:    quattro: >cinque sei< ⌈°( )°        ⌉
            four five six        |             |
326   SP:                        ⌊good ⌋ very good °lovely (.) nice°
327   I:    yeah bravo bravo
            well done well done
```

Both Ines and Ippolita are thus deliberately reinforcing the SPs' selection of the VoL, instead of systematically opting for the more widely documented operational mode of interpreted discourse, whereby feedback is omitted, especially when transparent.

Pauses

Sacks et al. (1974) distinguish between three types of discontinuities in talk: pauses, gaps and lapses. A *pause* is a silence which does not occur at a transition-relevance place, and, as such, is not perceived as a signal that the floor is made available to the next speaker. Whilst these pauses, which Hayashi (1996) calls "intraturn spaces", will be examined in the discussion of prosody (see 3.4), this paragraph will focus on inter-turn silences. When a silence arises at a TRP and another speaker self-selects for the next turn, the discontinuity is called a *gap*. Gaps can turn into *lapses*, that is extended spaces of non-talk, if no speaker is willing to take the floor. To avoid or resolve lapses, the current speaker may resume talking, thus transforming these silences into *pauses* separating two turns by the same speaker. For the sake of simplicity, all instances of discontinuities "between turns" have been subsumed here under the heading "pauses".

In the specific context of speech therapy, pauses may lose some of the connotations attached to them in ordinary conversation. When a pause occurs in place of the patient's answer, it rarely signals reluctance to respond to a question and is instead the manifestation of his health condition. As such, pauses are tolerated by the other participants, who do not exhibit signs of discomfort as is generally the case in everyday talk.

Linking these considerations back to the concept of adjacency trio, the following excerpt is offered as an example of an unmarked sequence displaying the pattern: SP's question — I's translation — SP's question. Sheila is asking Pino to name two sports items, thus implicitly selecting first the interpreter and then the patient as next speakers. In the absence of an answer by Pino, Sheila resolves the resulting pause by taking the floor again to reformulate the question:

```
[8]    T. 2  (228–233)
228  SP:  =°okay° (.) two things you could buy at a shop that sells things you need to play
229        sport
230  I:   °mhm° due cose che si possono compra:re in un nego:zio dove si ve:ndono (.)
           two things you can buy in a shop where they sell
231        eh:m arti:coli:: e – per quando uno deve andare a fare qualche tipo di sport
           items you can use when you practice some kind of sport
232        ((long pause))
233  SP:  what would you need to buy if you wanted to play cricket
```

As in smooth transitions, analysis of sessions 2 and 3 has also shown instances of marked as well as unmarked patterns, where it is the interpreter who steps in after a pause instead of the SP. In the following example, Ines breaks the patient's silence by rephrasing her translation of Sheila's original question. In self-selecting as next speaker, she displays the behaviour of a powerful participant, and the VoI merges once again with the VoM:

[9]   T. 2   (280–285)
280   SP: °mhm° what's a flower you could buy that has thorns
281   I: un tipo di fiore con le spine che lei potrebbe trovare da un vivaio come si chiama (.)
            a type of flower with thorns you can find at a nursery what is the name of
282   ques – una pianta con le spine che fa i fiori
            this a plant with thorns that has flowers
283   ((pause))
284   I: quella pianta che fa i fiori e che ha anche le spine
            that plant that has flowers and has thorns also
285   P: yeah=

The last example in this paragraph, which unlike all others is taken from T.1 and does not refer to a therapy session, portrays an interesting conversational exchange, where the VoI's operational mode is in full swing. Here the discontinuity is caused not by the patient's but by the interpreter's silence, in that Ines initially waits for Sheila to go on speaking. Sheila's intention, on the other hand, is to ease the interpreter's task by breaking down her utterance into chunks, a frequently observed feature in the conduct of primary speakers who are used to being interpreted, and a clear example of how they can implicitly acknowledge the requirements of the interpreting process. Paradoxically, however, this sensitivity clashes with a higher-level interpreting need, that of delaying one's translation until more of the message has been delivered. Consequently, as the pause lengthens and turns into a lapse, Ines resolves it not by translating, as the SP expects her to do, but by completing Sheila's sentence, thus urging her to take the floor again and add more information:

[10] T. 1   (73–81)
73   SP: =tomorrow (.) Luca (.) your son will go with you to the XXX[17]
74   ((pause))
75   I: and then you're meeting ⌐(there) ⌐
76   SP: ⌊ and   ⌋ I am sorry and I will meet you at the hospital=
77   I: =alright=
78   SP: =and be with you while the X-ray is being done
79   I: quindi doma:ni (.) quello che succederà è questo (.) l – la viene a prendere suo figlio (.) e la porta al
           so tomorrow what will happen is that your son will come to pick you up and take you to
80   XXX (.) all'ospedale voi due (.) Sheila invece sarà lì ad aspettarvi (.) e Sheila sarà con le:i mentre si fa
           hospital XXX you two Sheila instead will wait for you there and Sheila will stay with you while
81   il raggio (.) va bene↑
           the X-ray is being done okay

Overlaps

Except for back-channels, which for constraints of length will not be discussed in this section, relatively few instances of overlaps have emerged from the three transcripts. The following paragraph will illustrate the most significant ones, sorting them into three broad categories on the basis of their distance from TRPs.

Overlaps occurring *in the proximity of* a TRP were found to be brief, and were frequently the result of the interpreter's translation act, as in the following two excerpts, where Ines' right to the floor is acknowledged by the primary interlocutors' dropping out:

```
[11] T. 1 (165–167)
165  SP:   okay it's been organized    ⌈ °okay° ⌉
166  I:                                ⌊ hanno  ⌋ organizzato già è tutto apposto hanno già
                                         they have organised everything it's all right they have already
167         organizzato °va bene°↑
            organised okay

[12] T. 2 (107–110)
107  P:    ehm come si chiama l'altra:
           what's the other one called
108  I:    I'm not sure
109  P:    ehm non me lo ⌈ ricordo  ⌉
           I can't         | remember |
110  I:                  ⌊ what's   ⌋ the other one called altra >I can't remember
```

Emblematic of the SP's willingness to cede the floor is also excerpt [13]. Here the overlap takes place *at* a TRP, after a gap in the turn-taking sequence, when no one has been selected as next speaker. As the interpreter is waiting to hear more of the patient's utterance to be able to translate, the two primary interlocutors self-select simultaneously. By dropping out and letting the VoL speak — the patient is not so much providing an objective reason for the large variety of vegetables that he grows in his garden, as showing his pride in owning quite a substantial amount of land — Sheila is seen to adopt a non-directive interactional style:

```
[13] T. 2 (61–68)
61  SP:   oh (.) sounds like you have lots of variety
62  I:    pare che lei a — ha — una buona varietà (.) di cose una buona scelta
          it seems you have a wide variety of things a wide selection
63  P:    insomma
          well
64  SP:  ⌈⌈ what —
65  P:   ⌊⌊ avendo avendo tanta terra no
            when you have when you have a lot of land you know
66  I:    more or less I mean having a lot of s — land or soil
67  SP:   mhm °that helps° (.) what do you do to keep the snails (.) and birds (.) away from
68        the fruit and vegetables
```

Whilst the SP's behaviour may be a function of the specific activity being performed in the session, i.e. speech rehabilitation, it contrasts once again with the findings of other studies on interpreted medical encounters (see, for example, Englund Dimitrova 1997: 155–156) where doctors are found to take and maintain their turn regardless of the patient's attempt to claim it.

A second instance of simultaneous self-selection, this time involving a primary speaker and the interpreter, is the one illustrated in [14]. Here Ines translates Pino's correct answer and, following a short gap, takes the floor again to voice her favourable assessment, which comes to overlap with Sheila's feedback. The resulting pattern, P's answer — I's translation — I's assessment + SP's assessment, deviates from the unmarked adjacency trio described under point 2 above, and its interpretation can be similar to that of excerpts [2], [3] and [4].

```
[14] T. 2  (465–469)
465  I:    chi è e      ⌐ cosa fa
           who is it    │ what is she doing
466  P:                 └ è una lei è una donna
                          it's a she it's a woman
467  I:    it's a she it's a woman
468  SP:   ⌐⌐ °good°
469  I:    └└ mhm
```

The third group includes those instances of simultaneous talk which Nofsinger (1991: 102) calls "interruptions". Occurring *neither at nor near* a TRP, these overlaps violate the ordinary turn-taking mechanisms and are often considered as a threat to the current speaker's face. A rare example of interruption is shown in the following excerpt, where Sheila takes the floor during Ines' turn, to offer Pino a clue to the answer:

```
[15] T. 2  (284–289)
284  I:    quella pianta che fa i fiori e che ha anche le spine
           that plant that has flowers and has thorns also
285  P:    yeah=
286  I:    =eh   ⌐ qual è la pianta
                 │ what plant is it
287  SP:         └ A RO:::
288  I:    una ro:: (.) una pianta di ro:::
           a ro a plant of ro
289  P:    rose
```

Whilst it is possible that the SP intends thus to reaffirm her right to the floor, the overall tenor of the session would point to a different explanation. In her eagerness to help the patient, Sheila's disregard of the basic conversational rule that one party speaks at a time is evidence of an enthusiastic, high-involvement style, rather than an attempt at controlling the interaction.

3.2 Footing

With the analysis of footing, we move from sequences and turns to the participants' conversational alignments, which can coincide with an entire turn, but can also change within the same turn. Footing, as defined by Goffman (1981: 128), is "the alignment we take up to ourselves and the others present as expressed in the way we manage the production or reception of an utterance". Starting from the author's pioneering notion of "production format", with its distinction between the roles of "principal", "author" and "animator", Wadensjö (1998: 91–92) develops a parallel framework, which she calls "reception format", to account for three modes of listening and subsequent response, namely "responder", "recapitulator" and "reporter". In the present paragraph we will illustrate a model which, though inspired by Goffman's and Wadensjö's work, redefines some of these typologies, and integrates new ones.

Three considerations should serve as a point of departure for the following discussion. First, the model shown in Table 2 is a revised version of the classification used in our earlier studies (see note 3), where readers can find the frequency distribution of the different categories in the corpus of 32 interpreted sessions.[18] Second, the table should be viewed simply as an attempt to systematise a number of communicative occurrences, in full awareness that it does not reflect either the richness or the complexity of interactional scenarios. Third, the classification suggested here should be subjected to severe scrutiny by other researchers and, in particular, checked against further samples of authentic interpreted interaction.

With the exception of the category of principal, the model is constructed on the interconnection between the primary speaker's alignment to the other primary speaker and to the interpreter, and the latter's role as interlocutor or as addressed/unaddressed translator. Moving from the assumption that the footing of *reporter*[19] is the "unmarked" alignment — only in the sense that the interpreting scenario in which one party addresses the other directly and the interpreter uses the first person to identify in turn with each speaker is generally considered to be the canonical one — all the other categories can be conceived of, to a greater or lesser extent, as departures from it. Taking a distance from the utterance of the primary speaker, the interpreter may shift from the first to the third person, i.e. from the footing of reporter to that of *narrator*. Alternatively, she may want to signal commonality of purposes with the current speaker through the use of the first person plural, thus opting for the footing of *pseudo-co-principal*. When, on the other hand, the primary speaker addresses the interpreter to ask her to refer what s/he is saying to the other party, the interpreter's choice is between the two categories of *direct* and *indirect recapitulator*, i.e. between, once again, the first person, to bring the interlocutors closer together, and the third person, to maintain the distance between

Table 2. Categories of footing

Primary Speaker	Interpreter			FOOTING
	Initiator		Will you move over there, please?	PRINCIPAL
Who will take me there?	Interlocutor		The doctor will.	RESPONDER
(Tell her) I'll ask her some questions now.	Translator	addressed	Ora ti farò delle domande. *Now I will ask you some questions.*	DIRECT RECAPITULATOR
			(Dice che) ora ti farà delle domande. *(She says) she will ask you some questions.*	INDIRECT RECAPITULATOR
Now I'll ask you some questions.		unaddressed	Ora ti farò delle domande. *Now I will ask you some questions.*	REPORTER
			(Dice che) ora ti farà delle domande. *(She says) she will ask you some questions.*	NARRATOR
			Ora ti faremo delle domande. *Now we will ask you some questions.*	PSEUDO-CO-PRINCIPAL

them. As for the two remaining modes, which are farther away from the tenet of the interpreter's "invisibility", the footing of *principal* refers to the interpreter as initiator of a communicative act, whilst that of *responder* sees her relating as interlocutor to a primary speaker's utterance, which may or may not be explicitly addressed to her.

The following sections will illustrate the "marked" alignments which have been found in the transcripts. This means that, apart from the footing of reporter, which, though highly frequent, is the least interesting for the purpose of our discussion, the footings of direct and indirect recapitulator will also be excluded. The absence of these two categories runs counter to the predominant trends observed in the above-mentioned corpus, of which the three sessions are but a small portion, and is evidence of the atypical nature of these encounters, where primary speakers were seen to either speak directly to each other or interact with the interpreter as interlocutor. The incidence of the footing of principal, which will be exemplified first, is also noteworthy.

Principal

Leaving aside the interpreter's metalinguistic comments on the patient's utterances, which will be discussed in the section on additions (see 3.3), three cases will be illustrated here of autonomous interventions by Ines and Ippolita.

In the first sequence, Ines has just translated "bakery" with the Italian term "panificio", which contains the word the speech pathologist is trying to elicit from the patient, i.e. "pane", "bread". Realising that she has made the question easier for the patient and that she should have used instead the less telling synonym "fornaio", she feels she has to inform Sheila, and remains on this topic even after the latter has acknowledged the mishap and moves on to a new question. The effect of her protracted explanation — which can be read as a face-preserving act through self-criticism — is that the translation of the new question is delayed and the floor is repeatedly reassigned to the SP, who is thereby brought back to the interpreter's topic. Ines' decision to alert Sheila to the implications of her lexical choice is a manifestation of the concerns of the VoI, as excerpt [10] above was of its needs.

[16] T. 2 (355–374)
355   SP: °okay° (.) two things you could buy at a bakery
356   I: due cose che si possono comprare a — in un panificio
            two things you can buy at a breadshop
357   P: oh il pane
            bread
258   I: bread
359   SP: ⌈⌈mhm
360   I: ⌊⌊((addressing the speech pathologist)) **the word itself says it anyway so that**
361   **was a clue**
362   SP: yeah
363   I: ⌈⌈((laugh))
364   SP: ⌊⌊okay (.) what else can you buy at a bakery
365   I: °**breadshop you know**°
366   SP: ⌈⌈oh yeah fair enough yeah
367   I: ⌊⌊((laugh)) **that's the word in English**=
368   SP: =yeah=
369   I: **(it's) already used bakery I used the — the immediate term** yeah cos'altro allora il
                                                                          what else then
370   pa:ne e cos'altro (.) ((addressing the speech pathologist)) >°**yeah I should have**
            bread and what else
371   **used another word but anyway**°<
372   ((pause))
373   I: da un fornaio ((chuckle)) ((addressing the speech pathologist)) °**that's more**
            at the baker's
374   **bakery**° ((chuckle))

In the second sequence, Ippolita moves in the opposite direction. She takes off her interpreting hat and offers Sara some extra objects for the patient to identify. Seeing the interpreter's eagerness to help, the SP overcomes her initial reluctance:

```
[17] T. 3  (197–204)
197         ((the speech pathologist looks for other objects))
198  I:     ((addressing the speech pathologist)) °do you want — °
199  SP:    °no it's fine°=
200  I:     =something else↑
201  SP:    °no >it's alright<°
202  I:     I've got ⌈ props
203  SP:           ⌊ oh >that (sounds good)< (.) >props will be fine<
204  I:     ((the interpreter gives the speech pathologist a pen)) pen
```

An even more dramatic departure from a merely "echoic" role is shown in the third sequence. Here Ippolita tells the patient's wife, who is overly eager to answer on her husband's behalf, to go and sit at a distance. Without having been prompted to do so by the SP, she thus gives instructions for a more effective running of the therapy session. Since, judging from her words, the reason behind Ippolita's behaviour is not that her interpreting task might be disturbed, but rather that the patient might be "confused", the interpreter is seen here to adopt the authoritative VoM.

```
[18] T. 3  (14–21)
14   SP:   is your name Pietro
15   I:    il suo nome è Pietro↑
           is your name Pietro
16   SP:   yes: (.) or no
17   I:    ⌈ ⌈ sì o no↑       ⌉
18   W:   ⌊ ⌊ ma sì (.)      ⌟ yes ( )
              but of course
19   I:    signora lei si siede di là (.) per favore (.) altrimenti si confonde si siede di là (.)
           madam will you please sit there please otherwise he'll get confused sit over there
20         signora↑ (.) si siede di là
           madam sit over there
21   W:    ((addressing her husband)) risponda risponda sai↑ ((she moves away))
                       come on answer answer
```

Responder

Besides taking the initiative to make clarifications, offer help or give instructions, the interpreter is also frequently seen to respond directly to a primary interlocutor's utterance. This is a natural enough reaction when, for instance, she needs clarifications in order to translate accurately, as in the following excerpt, where Ines has difficulty understanding the Sicilian dialect spoken by Patrizio:

```
[19] T. 1  (113–116)
113  P:    ah ca a bocca ce l'ho piena di sti sti (scorco) tutta quanta murata di
           my mouth is full of these these it is all cemented with
```

114 I: **tutta quanta come**↑
            is it what
115 P: murata de scracchi lì (.) de a porcheria
            cemented with scum with rubbish
116 I: di porcheria in — in gola yeah but I feel that you know just my — my throat is full of gum
            (.)
            rubbish in the throat

or when the information has already been supplied by the other primary speaker earlier on in the encounter and the interpreter is simply reiterating it:

[20] T. 1 (153–154)
153 SP: I spoke to Rita this morning (.) **and she said that Luca could come**
154 I: Sheila ha parlato con Rita questa mattina e Rita ha detto che Luca può venire
            Sheila spoke with Rita this morning and Rita said that Luca can come

      (160–161)
160 P: appunto ma (alle sette) e mezza chi viene qua
            yes but at half past seven who is coming here
161 I: **chi:**↑ **Luca** (.) **Luca viene**
            who Luca Luca will come

or, clearly, when the interpreter is being personally addressed. In [21], as the session draws to a close, Patrizio, who has just been reassured by Ines that his son Luca will be present the following day at his X-ray, asks the interpreter when he will next see her. Ines' professional attitude is shown in her attentiveness to the SP's momentary exclusion from understanding, which she resolves by translating the patient's enquiry before answering it:

[21] T. 1 (182–184)
182 P: a lei quanno la vediamo
            when are we going to see you
183 I: **ehm io**↑ >when is he going to see me< **ehm mi ve::de ehm quando torna dall'ospedale il**
            me   *you'll see me when you come back from the*
            hospital
184   **pomeriggio o venerdì** (.) **mhm**↑
            in the afternoon or on Friday

A consequence of Ines' translation act is that the patient's VoL perspective is conveyed to the healthcare practitioner, instead of being judged by the interpreter as irrelevant and therefore not worth translating.[20]

Narrator

Highly frequent and equally natural is the interpreter's adoption of the footing of narrator in her translations of the SP's utterances. Differently from the trends observed in the larger corpus, where this alignment emerged as an attempt by the interpreter to separate her involved and sympathetic attitude from the therapist's

disaffiliative stance, in the three recorded sessions the interpreter's decision is simply dictated by the need to avoid ambiguity, as in the following excerpt, where Ines
is informing Patrizio that Sheila will take him to another hospital the next day:

[22] T. 1 (31–34)

31   SP: tomorrow morning (.) later tomorrow morning (.) I'm going to take you to the XXX

32   Hospital (.) for about half an hour

33   I: doma:ni verso metà matti:na (.) **Sheila** ((addressing the speech pathologist)) °you're going
             tomorrow around mid morning Sheila

34   too° ((the speech pathologist nods)) **Sheila** (.) **la porta** (.) **all'altro ospedale** (.) **il XXX** (.)
             Sheila will take you to the other hospital the XXX

The sequence, which justifies the patient's later question in [21] above, is also an
instance of an intra-turn shift in footing. Embedded in the translation is the role
of principal displayed by Ines as she seeks confirmation from Sheila of the correct-
ness of her statement.

A more interesting example is sequence [23], where Ines' explicit mention of
Sheila as the agent of the action she is narrating clearly conveys to the patient the
SP's caring attitude:

[23] T. 1 (56–58)

56   SP: I have even cooked some chocolate muffins to take up for you to try

57   I: **Sheila le ha preparato** (.) **una tarti:na** (.) **di cioccolata per dargliela domani** (.) **mhm**↑
             perfino
             Sheila has prepared a chocolate cake and she'll give it to you tomorrow mhm she has even

58   **questo ha fatto** ((soft chuckle))
             done this

The mode of narrator was recorded only once in the translations of the patient's
utterances — for which the footing of reporter was the norm — and appears to be
motivated by the patient's use of English in his reply to the SP's question. Thinking
that Sheila might not have understood Pino's unclear pronunciation, Ines instinc-
tively shifts to the third person, producing, in a lower voice, a sentence which
could be paraphrased as "He said he does not know":

[24] T. 2 (275–277)

275   P: I don't know ⌈(the name)⌉
276   SP: ⌊what's   ⌋ the type of flower=
277   I: =°**he wouldn't know**° un tipo di fiore mi dica
             a type of flower can you tell me

Once again the turn contains a double footing, given that the interpreter proceeds
to translate the SP's question as reporter.

Pseudo-co-principal

A more interesting, albeit rarer, mode is that of pseudo-co-principal, whereby the interpreter associates her identity with that of the SP, displaying the opposite attitude of the one described in the preceding paragraph. The following sequence is given as illustration:

[25] T. 3 (8–9)

8   SP: very good okay (.) u:mm I'm going to ask you some yes-or-no questions (.) °okay°↑
9   I: adesso **le facciamo** delle domande e: che lei deve rispondere col sì o col no
           now we will ask you some questions and you must answer yes or no

(311–312)

311 SP: °okay° (.) Pietro I'd like you to do some talking for me now
312 I: adesso signor Pietro **vogliamo** che: lei fa: – che parla (.) un pochettino
           now Mr. Pietro we would like you to do to speak a little

A last example of an odd intra-turn coexistence between the footings of narrator and pseudo-co-principal is offered in the following excerpt:

[26] T. 2 (403–406)

403 SP: °mhm° okay what I want you to do is tell me (.) >who you can see in the pictures<
404   (.) and what they are doing
405 I: quindi ora **Sheila vuole** che lei ci dica cosa vede: in queste imma:gini >in queste
           so now Sheila wants you to tell us what you see in these pictures in these
406   foto< e cosa stanno (.) face:ndo
           photographs and what they are doing

Here, the boundaries between the different voices become disorientingly blurred.

3.3 Divergent renditions: Additions

In the literature which investigates how interpreted — or "target" — texts may depart from source texts, the main focus has traditionally been on the performance of simultaneous interpreters, and on the analysis of omissions, additions and substitutions in terms of errors, sometimes even in contrast to the explicit purpose stated at the outset by the authors themselves (see Barik 1994).[21] However, more recent trends in the field have shifted attention towards a reading of these departures as "strategies". Kopczynski (1994) describes the survey he conducted on the attitudes and expectations displayed by conference speakers and audience towards the provision of interpreting services, including the preference for a more or less active role played by the interpreter. In other words (Kopczynski 1994: 93):

> [...] should s/he be the ghost of the speaker or should s/he intrude, i.e. omit, summarize or add portions of text? I suspect that the majority of speakers prefer the ghost role over that of the intruder. As bilingual and bicultural experts, however, we have a more or less conscious tendency to readjust or intrude.

Other authors stress not only the frequency, but also the advisability — under specific circumstances — of this intruder role. Analysing the function of additions in conference interpreting, Palazzi Gubertini (1998) points out that, clarity being the interpreter's main objective, there might be instances where the addition of material is necessary to explicate a potentially ambiguous original utterance. The same opinion is espoused by Falbo (1999), who distinguishes between "omission" and "loss", with the former being regarded as a deliberate choice. This perspective stems from two elements: on the one hand, the pivotal role attributed to the communicative goals of any one interpreted event (see Altman 1994), and, on the other, the influence of pragmatic factors, such as the situation and the recipients of the interpretation (see Kopczynski 1994; Viezzi 1996).

These contextual factors, which are undoubtedly significant in conference interpreting, are all the more crucial in face-to-face encounters. As a consequence, in this field, the departures from the speakers' original utterances acquire an additional value. As argued by Wadensjö (1998), the extent to which renditions relate to the preceding originals,[22] in terms of closeness versus divergence, allows for the understanding of the "potential interactional functions" performed by different kinds of interpreters' utterances (1998: 105).

In this section, an attempt will be made to explicate some of these functions. Given that omissions of information — Wadensjö's "zero renditions" (1998: 108) — and instances of substitution, namely semantic shifts, were rare and mostly insignificant occurrences, attention will be focused on additions. Four categories were identified, i.e. phatic, emphatic, explanatory and other.

With the exception of "phatic" additions, which are not treated as a separate group by other authors, the following categories were taken as a point of departure for our classification:

Barik's (1994: 125–126)

i.   *qualifier additions*, i.e. additions of a qualifier or a qualifying phrase absent in the original, for emphatic purposes;
ii. *elaboration additions*, i.e. additions in the form of an elaboration or any other straight addition to the text;

Cesca's (1997: 482– 493)

iii. *explanatory additions*, i.e. additions of elements in order to clarify the concept which is voiced;
iv. *emphatic additions*, aimed at stressing the content of the utterance;

Wadensjö's (1998: 107–108)

v. *expanded renditions*, which include more explicitly expressed information than the preceding original;
vi. *non-renditions*, i.e. texts which are analysable as an interpreter's initiative or response which does not correspond (as translation) to a prior original.

In the following discussion, "emphatic" additions will include instances largely corresponding to i. and iv., "explanatory" to ii., iii. and v., and "others" to vi. A preliminary consideration is, however, essential. Barik himself points out that what he calls qualifier and elaboration additions "refer essentially to the same event and could in fact be combined" (1994: 126). Similarly, the distinction between emphatic and explanatory additions is not always clear-cut and has therefore posed classification difficulties.

Phatic additions

The adjective "phatic", which stems from the Greek *phátis*, meaning "speech" (Bussmann 1996), was originally used by Malinowski in the phrase "phatic communion" to identify the social task of language, i.e. the creation of "ties of union" among individuals through the mere exchange of words (see Abercrombie 1994; Crystal 1992). The term has subsequently been borrowed — although with a slightly modified connotation — by Roman Jakobson, who defines as phatic one of the six basic functions of language,[23] namely the function performed in those messages "primarily serving to establish, to prolong, or to discontinue communication, to check whether the channel works [...], to attract the attention of the interlocutor or to confirm his continued attention" (Jakobson 1990: 75). As stressed by Altieri Biagi (1985: 352), the word "channel" not only suggests the physical medium, but can also be viewed as a metaphor to express the presence of an empathic attitude between interlocutors. Therefore, within the scope of this study the label "phatic" refers to those additions performing the dual function of back-channelling and reassuring tokens.

Analysis of the three transcripts has revealed that phatic additions are present only in the translations into Italian and that they serve two purposes. Firstly, they are used by interpreters to check whether patients have thoroughly understood the message, and as such they can be read as expressions of the VoI's need to monitor the effectiveness of the interpreter's role as "communicative channel". Secondly, they occur when potentially upsetting information is conveyed to the patient and are thus the expression of a "louder" VoL than the already caring one adopted by the SP.

The most frequent additions, which occur at the end of the information chunk and are often accompanied by a rising intonation, are the filler "mhm" — used as a request of agreement — and the expression "va bene" (all right). Only in a few cases does the interpreter use "vero" (true) and "giusto" (right). In [27], for instance, the SP wants Patrizio to understand that an X-ray is nothing to be afraid of:

[27] T. 1 (52–55)
52   SP: the X-ray is just like having an X-ray taken of your a:rm or your leg only it's your
53   neck
54   I: questi raggi sono come quelli che si fanno per un braccio o per una gamba **mhm**↑ solo che
           these rays are like those taken of an arm or a leg mhm it's just that
55   soltanto qui si fa alla gola
           only here it's taken of your throat

A few turns later, Patrizio is asked to try some mashed potato for lunch, so that his swallowing difficulty can be assessed. Since he first complains about it and then reluctantly accepts, Sheila underlines that he does not have to feel forced. The phatic addition, clearly aiming at soothing him, occurs twice:

[28] T. 1 (123–127)
123 SP: have a try: (.) if it's too difficult you don't have to have it all
124 I: ci prova
           have a try
125 P: ((cough))
126 I: ci prova **va bene**↑ poi se è troppo diffi:cile mangiare la patata allora la lasci (.) **va bene**↑
           have a try all right then if eating the potato is too hard just leave it all right
127 P: yeah va be'
           yeah okay

Emphatic additions

This category comprises repetitions of words, phrases or even whole sentences, as well as the use of synonyms belonging to the same level of formality, to stress a concept already mentioned — either in the same or in a preceding turn — without providing any further information. Instances of these additions, which, it must be stressed, are not used as a compensation strategy for a loss of information in a previous rendition, frequently feature in the translations into Italian, whilst they are absent in those into English.

Depending on the context, emphatic additions perform different functions. In some cases, they are the expression of the VoM encouraging the patient to respond. In [29], for instance, given the lack of an immediate and audible answer, it is Ippolita who speaks in this voice by repeating Sara's question three times (a similar example is shown in [9]):

[29] T. 3 (376–377)
376 SP: now I've got you talking ((she points to her watch)) what's this
377 I: ((pointing to the watch)) cos'è questo (.) **cos'è questo** (.) cos — (.) **cos'è::**↑
           what is this what is this wh- what is it

But the most striking instances are those in which the SP's selection of the VoL, in response to the patient's concerns, is further reinforced by the interpreter. In the following excerpt, Sheila is telling the patient that his temporary transfer to another hospital for an X-ray has already been arranged and that he does not need to worry about it. Seeing the patient's perplexity, the same concepts are repeated over and over by Ines a few turns later:

[30] T. 1 (155–159)
155 SP: don't worry about it the staff have already arranged with your fa:mily who will take you
156   everything is organized all you need to do is come along
157 I: non si preoccupi che qui:: (.) ehm le infermiere (.) hanno già parlato con la famiglia hanno
          don't worry because here the nurses have already talked to your family they have
158   già (.) fatto l'appuntamento tutto è apposto lei solo deve andare lì e la portano (.) mhm↑
          non
          already arranged the appointment everything is settled you just have to go there and they will
          take you mhm there're no
159   **ci son più problemi non si deve preoccupare di nient'altro**
          more problems you don't have to worry about anything else

          (165–170)
165 SP: okay it's been organized ⌈°okay°⌉
166 I: ⌊hanno⌋ organizzato già è **tutto apposto hanno già**
                                    they have organised everything it's all right they have already
167   **organizzato** °va bene°↑
          organised okay
168 SP: they have worked something out
169 I: sono arrivati a — a qualcosa mhm↑ **a qualche decisio::ne si sono messi d'acco::rdo quindi**
          per
          they have reached so- something some kind of decision they found an agreement so for
170   **domani è apposto**
          tomorrow it's settled

The passage allows for similar comments to those made for [27] and [28]: the VoL, carried here by the over-repetition, is once again aimed at reassuring Patrizio. Evidence of their analogous function is the presence in this sequence of phatic additions, namely the filler "mhm" and the expression "va bene".

Explanatory additions

As pointed out by Mishler (1984: 172), in a medical encounter the only participant who is usually competent in both the VoM and the VoL is the professional, who has to decide whether or not to convert patients' lifeworld utterances into medical terms, and medical issues into lifeworld terms. In an interpreted medical encounter, this decision may be taken at a second level, if healthcare practitioners do not make code adjustments and interpreters do so in their stead, by adding information aimed at clarifying a message which they consider to be potentially obscure for the patient.

As was the case for the first two categories, explanatory additions were recorded almost exclusively in the translations for the patient. The pattern is rather straightforward: the literal translation of a word or phrase is followed either by the explanation of its meaning, or by a synonym belonging to a more informal level of language, as in the following example:

[31] T. 1 (46–51)
46   SP: while we're at the XXX (.) I will give you some food and some drink (.) then we will
47   take an X-ray of your throat (.) so that I can watch (.) if the food and drink goes the right
48   way to the stomach (.) or the wrong way to the chest
49   I: sì quindi domani mentre le fanno i raggi (.) **prende una foto un raggio da questa parte della**
           yes so tomorrow while they're taking the X-ray she takes a photo a ray from this side of the
50   **faccia** per vedere la gola mentre le danno da mangia::re e un po' da bere così riesce poi a
           face to see the throat while they're giving you to eat and something to drink so that then Sheila can
51   vedere Sheila se va dalla parte giusta o se va dall'altra parte che non deve andare
           see whether it goes the right way or the other way where it doesn't have to go

Since the term "X-ray" is perceived as a possible source of perplexity, Ines resorts to a paraphrase, describing it as a photo. In other words, she translates not only English into Italian, but also the technical term into a language which is easily accessible to the patient. This trend, commonly found in the larger corpus, does not often figure in the three transcribed sessions, for two reasons: firstly, two out of the three encounters are therapy sessions, in which the SP is making reference to everyday activities and objects, and wants the patient to practice basic vocabulary and syntactic structures; secondly, it has repeatedly been stressed that both Sheila and Sara display an involved attitude, which manifests itself through their extensive use of the VoL.

Other additions

This category includes those instances which Wadensjö calls "non-renditions" (1998: 108), namely interpreter's utterances lacking a corresponding original. Based on their main functions, such instances can be subdivided into seven groups, four of which (points 1 to 4 below) are also mentioned in the *Guide to Good Practice*, published by the *British Association of Community Interpreters* in 1989 and cited by Leonor Zimman (1993: 219). With the exception of categories 6 and 7, all others are the expression of the VoI's operational needs.

Adopting the footings of principal and responder as discussed in 3.2, interpreters may take the initiative to:

1.   *ask for clarification if the concept voiced by one interlocutor has not been clearly heard or thoroughly understood*: an illustration of this are examples [19] line

114, and [33] line 74. Given that all three patients are affected by speech impairments, this was a frequent occurrence in all analysed sessions;

2. *point out if a client has not understood the message despite the correct rendition.* No examples have been found in the three sessions, although a few instances of this category were recorded in the larger corpus;

3. *alert a client to a possible missed inference,* as shown in the following sequence:

[32] T. 2 (246–253)
246 SP: two things you could buy at (.) a nursery
247 I: due co:se che: uno troverebbe da un vivaio (.) sa cos'è un vivaio↑
           two things you could find at a nursery do you know what a nursery is
248 P: ye:s
249 I: ((addressing the speech pathologist)) **sometimes the (.) the te:rms in Italian are no**
250   **longer** ⌐ **(used)** ((chuckle))=
251 SP: └ oka:y ((soft chuckle))
252 I: =**they adopt the English one he's all right with that**↑ ((turning to the patient)) da
253   un vivaio allora che cosa possiamo trovare
           at a nursery then what can we find

Ines is not sure whether Pino is familiar with the Italian word for nursery, i.e. "vivaio", given that it is not uncommon to see first-generation immigrants using expressions of the local languages in place of their native tongue equivalents. Therefore, she first ascertains whether the patient has understood the term, and proceeds to explain to Sheila the reason for her intervention;

4. *ask a client to modify his/her delivery in order to accommodate the interpreting process,* as exemplified in [10] line 75, where Ines asks Sheila to complete the sentence before translating it;

5. *comment on their renditions,* as in [16];

6. *answer in the first person when directly addressed by one interlocutor,* as in [21];

7. *offer help,* as in [17], *give instructions,* as in [18], and *provide metalinguistic explanations of the client's utterances.* Given that the latter is a distinctive feature of interpreting in speech pathology, the following sequence is offered as an example among many:

[33] T. 2 (73–85)
73 P: (per le lumanchi) usi:: il veleno
         (for the snails) you use the poison
74 I: come scusi↑
         pardon
75 P: per le lumache
         for the snails
76 I: per le lumache↑ mhm
         for the snails mhm
77 P: gli (metto) il veleno
         I put the poison

```
78   I:    mhm I put the poison for the (.) snails and the word snail camed re — came really
79         mumbled at first I wasn't able to grasp it=
80   SP:   =mhm
81   I:    but then the second time he said it it was=
82   SP:   fixed
83   I:    yes    ┌it was=
84   SP:          └okay
85   I:    =fixed yeah
```

As already emphasised in the introductory paragraph to the present work, the description of the patient's speech enables the SP to assess his progress and provide appropriate feedback, as shown in the continuation to the above sequence:

[34] T. 2 (86–87)
```
86   SP:   it's good that when (.) you said the word snail and it wasn't clear (.) you could fix
87         it yourself and say it again better
```

3.4 Prosody

Analysis of prosody — the term is used here in its broader meaning to refer to suprasegmental features of speech — will consider three aspects: speech rate, sound duration and loudness. When discussing pauses in turn-taking, passing mention was made of "intraturn spaces". As Hayashi (1996) observes, these brief silences, or unfilled pauses, may be due to a variety of factors, such as loss of words, distraction, hesitation, but also empathic involvement. Examples of the latter function abound in our transcripts, where the SP is frequently seen to slow down elocution. This is achieved not only through the insertion of pauses between and within intonational phrases, but also through the lengthening of vowel sounds, as in the following utterances:

[35] T.2 (177)
```
177  SP:   I want you to tell me (.) two things (.) that you could bu::y in (.) a hardware shop
```

```
     (391–392)
391  SP:   sometimes when (.) you're ta::lking (.) you know what you want to say but you
392        don't give enough (.) information (.) to repeat while we're listening
```

Whilst a slower speech rate is a common enough way to make utterances clearer and more easily understandable to elderly patients, especially patients with speech disorders, the SP's selection of this pattern is a consequence of her addressing the patient directly and speaking to him as naturally as if no interpretation were needed. Her attention to the patient's difficulties is emulated by the interpreters, who display the same prosodic behaviour in their translations, as shown in the following lines which continue the previous example:

[36] T.2 (393–396)

393 I: delle volte: quando uno si trova (.) parlando (.) uno (.) sa quello che vuole dire
           sometimes when one is speaking one knows what he wants to say
394   però (.) il modo in cui viene fuo:ri è ⌈non c'è abbas – =
           but the way it comes out is |*there isn't enough*
395 P: ⌊°yeah yeah°
396 I: =l'informazio:ne che lei ha dato non è sufficiente=
           the information you have given is not enough

The interpreters' tuning in to the speech pathologists' overall conversational style goes beyond a mere echoic behaviour and results in their independent adoption of the same prosodic patterns, even when these are absent in the immediately preceding original utterances, as shown in excerpts [1] lines 189–190 (intra-turn pauses) and [2] lines 92–93 (lengthened vowels).

The very last example which concludes our analysis of the participants' voices is offered as an attempt to convey at least a glimpse of the relaxed atmosphere that characterised the encounters. Here, as in [15] line 287, a traditional indicator of a dominant verbal behaviour, loudness, loses all connotations of aggressiveness and becomes the index of a high-involvement style:

[37] T.1 (144–147)

144 P: no wanna no wanna quiddi taliani
           they don't want they don't want Italians
145 I: ah:: they don't want Italian ones there↑ ((laugh))
146 SP: ((amused tone of voice)) they take ⌈A:NYONE there   ⌉
147 I: ⌊((wholehearted laugh))   ⌋ chiu:nque può andare lì
           ((chuckle))
                                                                           anyone can go there

4. Conclusions

The study of interpreting conduct reported in this paper has revealed patterns of interaction whose complexity can hardly be described in terms of a voice simply "echoing", in turns, each of the other two. The concept of the "voice of interpreting" proposed here has emerged as a polyphonic and shifting variable, which was locally determined by the interpreters' perception of their own and the other participants' needs and orientations to the unfolding activity. Besides the numerous metalinguistic explanations of the patients' utterances, which are the more manifest instances of the interpreter's semantic autonomy and derive from the specific "activity system" (Bolden 2000: 415) characterising speech therapy, all of the three sessions have shown evidence of the interpreter's pronounced involvement in the interaction. This was seen as taking many forms: from her sharing in the speech pathologist's control of turn-taking and topic development, to her adopting the footings of principal, responder and, occasionally, pseudo-co-principal, to her making phatic, emphatic and explanatory additions and slowing down elocution for the benefit of the patient.

When read in the light of the chosen theoretical framework, these forms of conduct are seen to express a meaning and significance that we have attempted to explicate, albeit in a fragmented manner, in the successive layers of our analysis, and that will be recomposed here in a more organic vision. Taking as a point of departure Mishler's description of voice in terms of functions of specific features of discourse, we have observed in all three sessions a clear predominance of the voice of the lifeworld, brought about not only by the SPs' frequent "translation" of the voice of medicine "into patients' terms" (Mishler 1984: 172), but by a second act of translation, this time of an inter-lingual nature, on the part of the interpreter. In other words, the latter's display of an interactionally powerful role, which at times took on the tones of authoritativeness characteristic of the VoM and at other times reflected the operational mode of the VoI, was encapsulated in her overall tendency to strengthen, by means of her competence in the patient's language, the healthcare practitioner's empathic model of communication.

The dynamics observed in the current study, where the medical providers were willing to cede the floor to both interpreter and patient, were open to the patients' concerns, and were ready to reassure and encourage them, are not representative of the findings of our earlier investigations (see note 3), where the translation of the VoM into the VoL generally occurred at the interpreting stage only. Underlying this minority medical practice is an ideal which has silently run through the entire paper and which, despite the descriptive nature of our research project, we have no difficulty in acknowledging as ours, the ideal of "humane medical care". Referring one last time to Mishler's work where he writes (1984: 185):

> [...] it is clear that strengthening the voice of the lifeworld promotes both humaneness and effectiveness of care. The critical question is: How can the voice of the lifeworld be strengthened?

a partial answer to his question was given in this paper, where the creation of a relaxed and uninhibiting atmosphere was shown to be the product of a joint effort. In the specific circumstances of our sessions, where the patients' speech disorders necessarily limited their contribution to the interaction, this effort was made principally by the healthcare practitioner and the interpreter. Even in T.1, where the patient's ability to communicate was less severely impaired, the spontaneity of his remarks and the frequency of his questions were clearly encouraged by the attitudes of his interlocutors, although he was never found to actively share in their mirth. Whilst transcriptions might help researchers detect patterns that would otherwise escape attention owing to the evanescence of the oral medium, only by listening to the audio-tapes and, even more, by being physically present can this atmosphere be fully appreciated. And this is precisely what we witnessed in the three encounters, thanks not only to the personalities of both the healthcare and interpreting professionals, but also to the latter's understanding of their role as "communicators", rather than "just translators".

As Wadensjö (1998: 284) points out, "primary parties are dependent on the interpreter's involvement in interaction to be able to contribute in their own right to a certain communicative atmosphere". This means that strict adherence to a dry, formal, passive and detached interpreting style, though it might be in line with an idealised notion of professional conduct, is not always the best way to serve one's clients, especially when their intention is to engage in a friendly and co-operative dialogue. Dialogue being an intrinsically relational activity, it would seem reasonable that "dialogue interpreters" should select their communication strategies on the basis of the relational models which characterise a given interaction. It is therefore a fortunate coincidence that the etymology of the term "dialogue" should point in that direction, as one of the meanings of the Greek verb *légein* is precisely "to choose", "to select".

Notes

1. Although this paper is the outcome of a joint research project carried out by the two authors, Sections 1.2, 2, 3.1, 3.2 and 4 were written by Raffaela Merlini, and Sections 1.1, 3.3 and 3.4 by Roberta Favaron.

2. The National Accreditation Authority for Translators and Interpreters (NAATI) was established by the Australian federal and state governments in 1977 and entrusted with the tasks of setting professional standards, developing and implementing accreditation procedures and approving interpreting and translation courses (Ozolins 1998: 40).

3. The 32 interpreted encounters were observed over a five-month period, from March through July 2001, in a number of Melbourne's healthcare facilities, including general hospitals, rehabilitation clinics, mental health centres, nursing homes and patients' houses. Since recording of most of the encounters (29 out of 32) was not allowed, the observation process was systematised through the use of an "observation sheet", containing a set of preselected parameters partly borrowed from systemic functional linguistics, which had to be filled in before, during and soon after the sessions. The results of this earlier investigation can be found in Merlini & Favaron (2003), Favaron (2004) and Merlini (2005).

4. For the purpose of straightforward identification with their roles, patients have been given fictitious names beginning with the letter "P", speech pathologists' names beginning with the letter "S", and interpreters with the letter "I". Moreover, to facilitate cross-referencing with the data contained in Favaron (2004), where the observational study is amply illustrated (see note 3), the interpreters' names have not been changed.

5. A research project run by Raffaela Merlini at the University of Macerata, Italy, is under way to build a corpus of recorded dialogue interpreting sessions in a variety of fields, including health-care practice and immigration services. The long-term view is to integrate a quantitative per-spective, once the corpus has acquired meaningful dimensions.

6. Habermas (1970) makes a distinction between two "modes of consciousness", the "techno-cratic", which is oriented to technical rules and transforms lifeworld problems into technical ones, and the "symbolic" expressed through ordinary language. In his view, the domination of the technocratic consciousness and the absorption of ordinary language by technical language lead to the distortion and suppression of human values.

7. Universality, affective neutrality and functional specificity are, according to Parsons (1951), the basic norms that underlie role relationships between patients and physicians.

8. In her insightful article on interpreters' involvement in history taking, Bolden (2000) uses Mishler's concept of the "voice of medicine" to show how medical interpreters can share the physicians' orientation towards obtaining objectively formulated and decontextualized descrip-tions of patients' symptoms.

9. In the remaining discussion, interpreters and doctors will be conventionally referred to as "she" and patients as "he".

10. Fairclough (1992: 138) engages here in a dialogue with Mishler (1984), from whom he takes the transcript of the medical interview in question, and elaborates on his dialectic representa-tion of the interaction between the "voice of medicine" and the "voice of the lifeworld".

11. Conversationalists are able to detect a TRP through such signals as the end of a syntactic unit, pauses, changes in intonation and volume of voice, and kinesics.

12. Englund Dimitrova (1993) shows how some of the principles for turn-taking put forward by Sacks et al. (1974) do not apply to interpreted interaction. She mentions in particular principle 5 about non-fixed speaker order, a principle which is invalidated by the need for the interpreter to take a turn every other turn.

13. The term "trio" has been purposely chosen to convey both the general meaning of "group of three things" and, in a figurative sense, the reference to a performance by "three voices".

14. Examples are numbered consecutively. The acronyms T. 1, T. 2 and T. 3 identify the tran-script from which a given excerpt has been taken, whilst the numbers in parentheses refer to the place of the reported lines in the transcript. For easier reference, the latter also appear beside each line. Idiomatic translations into English of the Italian utterances are shown in italics. Fea-tures of interest are shown in bold.

15. A much more extensive and questionable presence of this marked pattern is recorded by Bolden (2000: 393). In her study, the interpreter is frequently seen to proceed from a doctor-initiated question through an independent questioning sequence, which is then summarised for the doctor's benefit.

16. Englund Dimitrova (1997: 160) observes that the non-interpretation of feedback signals may be a deliberate strategy, since the interpreter might not perceive the feedback as an informa-tion-carrying part of the communication.

17. The 3 X's replace the name of the hospital.

18. It should be noted that in the earlier version of our model, the footing of principal also included those instances which are grouped here under responder. Moreover, the footings of recapitulator (a) and (b) have been renamed as "direct" and "indirect".

19. The mode of reporter outlined here goes beyond the restricted sense indicated by Wadensjö (1998: 93) of "animator" — which, as she rightly says, cannot apply to interpreting given the necessary production of linguistically different versions of the original utterances — and includes the notion of "author". As a result, the mode of recapitulator itself takes on new contours.

20. The opposite behaviour is recorded by Bolden (2000: 423–414), as she finds that patients' contextualized and subjective accounts are consistently dismissed and excluded from the interpreter's translations for the doctor.

21. Barik (1994 [1971]) created a "coding system" to classify how interpreters may omit, add or substitute material uttered by speakers, considering only the latter as a possible "error" and ruling out any attempt at evaluation; nevertheless, his system has crucially influenced subsequent research on *quality* in interpretation.

22. Following Wadensjö's terminology, a "rendition" is "a stretch of text corresponding to an utterance voiced by an interpreter", whereas "originals" are "all utterances voiced by primary interactants" (1998: 106).

23. A brief overview of Jakobson's model of the speech event is deserving of note: "Jakobson [...] began to explore language as an interpersonal means of communication and developed his theory of the interrelation between the speech event and the functions of language. He argued that there are six factors of the speech event: speaker, addressee, code (language system), message (individual language usage), contact (means by which the message is transmitted), context — and that a predominance of focus on one of those factors determines one of the six major functions of language: emotive/expressive, conative (appeal-function), metalinguistic, poetic, phatic and referential, respectively." (Waugh 1994).

References

Abercrombie, D. (1994). Phatic communion. In R. E. Asher (Ed.), *The encyclopedia of language and linguistics*. Vol. 6. Oxford/New York/Seoul/Tokyo: Pergamon Press.

Altieri Biagi, M. L. (1985). *Linguistica essenziale*. Milano: Garzanti.

Altman, J. (1994). Error analysis in the teaching of simultaneous interpreting: A pilot study. In S. Lambert & B. Moser-Mercer (Eds.), *Bridging the gap: Empirical research in simultaneous interpretation*. Amsterdam/Philadelphia: Benjamins, 25–38.

Atkinson, J. M. & Heritage, J. (Eds.) (1984). *Structures of social action: Studies in conversation analysis*. Cambridge: Cambridge University Press.

Barik, H. C. (1994). A description of various types of omissions, additions and errors of translation encountered in simultaneous interpretation. In S. Lambert & B. Moser-Mercer (Eds.), *Bridging the gap: Empirical research in simultaneous interpretation*. Amsterdam/Philadelphia: Benjamins, 121–137 [First published in *META* 16 (4), 199–210, 1971].

Bolden, G. (2000). Toward understanding practices of medical interpreting: Interpreters' involvement in history taking. *Discourse Studies* 2 (4), 387–419.

Bussmann, H. (1996). *Routledge dictionary of language and linguistics*. Translated and edited by G. P. Trauth and K. Kazzazi. London/New York: Routledge.

Cesca, D. (1997). *Madrelingua versus non-madrelingua: studio sperimentale in interpretazione simultanea russo-italiano*. Unpublished thesis, SSLMIT, University of Trieste.

Critchley, M. (Ed.) (1978). *Butterworths medical dictionary*. London: Butterworths.

Crystal, D. (1992). *An encyclopedic dictionary of language and languages*. Oxford/Cambridge: Blackwell.

Drew, P. & Heritage, J. (Eds.) (1992). *Talk at work. Interaction in institutional settings*. Cambridge: Cambridge University Press.

Eggins, S. & Slade, D. (1997). *Analysing casual conversation*. London/Washington: Cassell.

Englund Dimitrova, B. (1993). Turntaking in interpreted discourse: Interplay of implicit and explicit rules. In K. Cankov (Ed.), *Problemi na sociolingvistikata. Ezikovata situacija v mikro- i makrosocialnite obstnosti*. Veliko Târnovo: Universitetsko izdatelstvo, 15–21.

Englund Dimitrova, B. (1997). Degree of interpreter responsibility in the interaction process in community interpreting. In S. E. Carr, R. Roberts, A. Dufour & D. Steyn (Eds.), *The Critical Link: Interpreters in the community*. Amsterdam/Philadelphia: Benjamins, 147–164.

Fairclough, N. (1992). *Discourse and social change*. Cambridge: Polity Press.

Falbo, C. (1999). Analisi degli errori: obiettivi, problemi, prospettive. In M. Viezzi (Ed.), *Quality forum 1997*. Trieste: SSLMIT, 73–80.

Favaron, R. (2004). *L'interprete ai raggi X*. Trieste: EUT.

Fele, G. (1999). L'analisi della conversazione come una sociologia particolare. In R. Galatolo & G. Pallotti (Eds.), *La conversazione. Un'introduzione allo studio dell'interazione*. Milano: Raffaello Cortina Editore, 23–42.

Frankel, R. (1990). Talking in interviews: A dispreference for patient-initiated questions in physician-patient encounters. In G. Psathas (Ed.), *Interaction competence*. Lanham, MD: University Press of America, 231–262.

Gentile, A., Ozolins, U. & Vasilakakos, M. (1996). *Liaison interpreting. A handbook*. Melbourne: Melbourne University Press.

Goffman, E. (1981). *Forms of talk*. Oxford: Blackwell.

Habermas, J. (1970). *Toward a rational society*. Boston, MA: Beacon Press.

Hayashi, R. (1996). *Cognition, empathy and interaction: Floor management of English and Japanese conversation*. Norwood, NJ: Ablex.

Jackson, C. A. (1988). Linguistics and speech–language pathology. In F. J. Newmeyer (Ed.), *Language: Psychological and biological aspects*, vol. 3 of *Linguistics: The Cambridge survey*. Cambridge/New York/Port Chester/Melbourne/Sydney: Cambridge University Press, 256–273.

Jakobson, R. (1990). *On language*. Ed. by L. R. Waugh & M. Monville-Burston. Cambridge/London: Harvard University Press.

Kopczynski, A. (1994). Quality in conference interpreting: Some pragmatic problems. In S. Lambert & B. Moser-Mercer (Eds.), *Bridging the gap: Empirical research in simultaneous interpretation*. Amsterdam/Philadelphia: Benjamins, 87–99.

Langdon, H. W. & Cheng, L. L. (2002). *Collaborating with interpreters and translators. A guide for communication disorders professionals*. Eau Claire, Wisconsin: Thinking Publications.

Langdon, H. W. (2002). *Interpreters and translators in communication disorders. A practitioner's handbook*. Eau Claire, Wisconsin: Thinking Publications.

Merlini, R. & Favaron, R. (2003). Community interpreting: Re-conciliation through power management. *The Interpreters' Newsletter* 12, 205–229.

Merlini, R. (2005). Alla ricerca dell'interprete ritrovato. In M. Russo & G. Mack (Eds.), *Interpretazione di trattativa. La mediazione linguistico-culturale nel contesto formativo e professionale*. Milano: Hoepli, 19–40.

Mishler, E. G. (1984). *The discourse of medicine: Dialectics of medical interviews*. Norwood, NJ: Ablex.

Nofsinger, R. E. (1991). *Everyday conversation*. Newbury Park: Sage Publications.

Ozolins, U. (1998). *Interpreting and translating in Australia: Current issues and international comparisons*. Melbourne: Language Australia.

Palazzi Gubertini, M. C. (1998). Des ajouts en interpretation. Pourquoi pas? *The Interpreters' Newsletter* 8, 135–149.

Parsons, T. (1951). *The social system*. New York: Free Press.

Roy, C. B. (1996). An interactional sociolinguistic analysis of turn-taking in an interpreted event. *Interpreting* 1 (1), 39–67.

Sacks, H., Schegloff, E. A. & Jefferson, G. (1974). A simplest systematics for the organization of turn-taking in conversation. *Language* 50 (4), 696–735.

Schegloff, E. A. & Sacks, H. (1973). Opening up closings. *Semiotica* 8 (4), 289–327.

Schegloff, E. A. (1992). On talk and its institutional occasions. In P. Drew & J. Heritage (Eds.), *Talk at work. Interaction in institutional settings*. Cambridge: Cambridge University Press, 101–136.

Silverman, D. (1987). *Communication and medical practice*. London: Sage.

Sinclair, J. McH. & Coulthard, M. (1975). *Towards an analysis of discourse: The English used by teachers and pupils*. Oxford: Oxford University Press.

Viezzi, M. (1996). *Aspetti della qualità in interpretazione*. S.eR.T. 2. Trieste: SSLMIT.

Wadensjö, C. (1998). *Interpreting as interaction*. London/New York: Longman.

Waugh, L. R. (1994). Jakobson, Roman (1896–1982). In R. E. Asher (Ed.), *The encyclopedia of language and linguistics*. Vol. 6. Oxford/New York/Seoul/Tokyo: Pergamon Press.

Zimman, L. (1993). Intervention as a pedagogical problem in community interpreting. In C. Dollerup & A. Lindegaard (Eds.), *Teaching translation and interpreting 2*. Amsterdam: Benjamins, 217–224.

Appendix: Transcription key

Symbols		Meaning
A ⌐⌐ well I said B LL Yes		utterances starting simultaneously
A she's ⌐right ⌐ B L huh mm ⌐		overlapping utterances
A I agree= B =me too		latched utterances
(.)		untimed pause within a turn
((pause))		untimed pause between turns
↑		rising intonation
wo:::rd		lengthened vowel or consonant sound
word – word		abrupt cut-off in the flow of speech
<u>word</u>		emphasis
WORD		increased volume
°word°		decreased volume
>word<		quicker pace
((word))		relevant contextual information; characterisations of the talk; vocalisations that cannot be spelled recognisably
(word)		transcriber's guess
( )		unrecoverable speech

Fillers		Meaning
English	*Italian*	
umm	umm	doubt
mhm	mhm	expression or request of agreement
ah	ah; eh	emphasis
eh	eh	query
uh	ehm	staller
oh	oh	surprise

BOOK REVIEWS

Carmen Valero Garcés and Guzmán Mancho Barés (Eds.). *Traducción
e interpretación en los servicios públicos: Nuevas necesidades para nuevas
realidades / Community Interpreting and Translating: New Needs for New
Realities*. Alcalá: Universidad de Alcalá, Servicio de Publicaciones, 2002.
279 pp. ISBN 84-8138-490-9.

Carmen Valero Garcés (Ed.). *Traducción e interpretación en los servicios
públicos. Contextualización, actualidad y futuro*. Granada: Comares,
2003. XII + 298 pp. ISBN 84-8444-686-7. [Interlingua 39.]

Reviewed by Holly Mikkelson

This review encompasses both a CD containing the proceedings of the Fifth International Conference on Translation and the First National Conference on Translation and Interpretation in Public Services, held in Alcalá de Henares, Spain, in
February 2002; and a follow-up book with articles, essays and interviews on community interpreting.

I. Proceedings on CD (Valero Garcés & Mancho Barés, Eds.)

The CD is a manifestation of the latest trend in publications, providing materials
in electronic form rather than hard copy. This format offers several advantages:
The reader can print out only the articles that are of special interest at a given moment; it is easier to search and navigate through the proceedings, allowing for a
specific term or concept to be researched throughout the volume; storage is much
more compact; and dissemination of the materials is much more efficient (though
this raises copyright concerns for the authors, who may fear rampant unauthor-
ized copying of their work).

The CD is accompanied by a printed booklet containing abstracts of all the
articles, in both Spanish and English, thereby making it possible for the reader to
decide which ones to select and read in their entirety. The articles themselves are
in either English or Spanish, without translations, so if people who do not read
Spanish are intrigued by the English abstract of an article written in Spanish, they
may be disappointed at not being able to actually read it (but at least they will
know what they are missing!). The articles are organized into five sections: (1) an
introduction by the editors, (2) guest contributions by two leaders in the field of

community interpreting, (3) papers on community interpreting in Spain, (4) papers on community interpreting in other countries, and (5) articles on the professionalization of translation and interpreting in general.

It would be helpful if the abstracts in the printed booklet indicated the page numbers of the articles on the CD so that the reader would not have to return to the table of contents each time to find a given paper. The files on the CD are in PDF format, so the reader must be familiar with the search and navigation features of that program to take full advantage of the CD format.

As is typical of conference proceedings, there is some lack of cohesiveness among the papers, which cover whatever topics the presenters chose to discuss within the overarching theme of the conference. Thus, some provide a broad view of a general issue and others focus very narrowly on a single language, location or problem. There does seem to be a uniform style and format, however, which is to the credit of the editors. Some of the contributions do not seem particularly relevant to community interpreting and translating, especially those in the final section on professionalization. For example, the paper on audiovisual translation, while interesting, might be better placed in a volume on multimedia translation and interpreting.

The guest contributors, Ann Corsellis and Helge Niska, are internationally recognized experts who have written extensively on community interpreting. Corsellis's paper, "Creating a Professional Context for Public Service Interpreters and Translators," presents an overview of the steps each country should take to make community interpreting a viable profession. Niska's paper, "Introduction to Terminology and Terminology Tools," is much narrower in focus. Although terminology is certainly an essential element of any type of interpreting and should be given more attention in interpreter training programs, it is frankly hard to see why this work is featured so prominently at the beginning of the proceedings. It would fit better among the third category of papers covering various topics relevant to translating and interpreting in public services.

The next series of contributions, on community interpreting in Spain, provides useful insights and information about the work of translators and interpreters in specific settings such as the courts and police stations, in specific languages such as a signed language and Moroccan Arabic, and in specific parts of Spain such as the Canary Islands. The papers in this part also deal with more general issues, such as the role of the community interpreter and interpreter training.

Researchers and practitioners from around the world offer their perspectives on a wide variety of topics in the next section of the proceedings. Again, there is considerable variation in the breadth and depth of the pieces, as evidenced by Jan Cambridge's analysis of "Interlocutor Roles and the Pressures on Interpreters" and

Mette Rudvin's article on "Cross-Cultural Aspects of Community Interpreting in Italy," at one end of the continuum and Mora Morelli's work on interpreting for homeless people and María del Carmen Riddel's contribution on the impact that living in exile has on the discourse of immigrant writers, at the other extreme. The papers examine interpreting in specific settings such as hospitals and courts, aspects of interpreter training, and issues of applied linguistics.

The final section, as noted above, is a collection of contributions on the professionalization of translation and interpreting, some of them tangentially related to community interpreting (such as studies of legal German and English) and some not really relevant, but interesting to read anyway. Their presence in this volume can be justified on the grounds that community interpreters do need to be aware of matters such as assessing quality in translation and parliamentary interpreting in order to be well-rounded professionals.

II. Follow-up book (Valero Garcés, Ed.)

As explained in the prologue, this volume is a follow-up on the proceedings of the 2002 conference reviewed here, however the focus is exclusively on Spain. Moreover, all of the papers are published in Spanish (some of them translations from English), making the materials accessible to a new audience. The corollary, of course, is that they are not available to anyone who does not read Spanish; but in any case many of the international contributors have also published in English elsewhere. It would be useful to have English translations of the articles on public service interpreting in Spain; perhaps this would be a good project for some translation students.

Although there is considerable overlap between this book and the conference proceedings in terms of the subjects covered and even some of the contributors, the articles compiled here provide an update on the situation a year later and go into more depth on many issues. This work represents a tremendous effort on the part of the editor, who had to compile the writings of dozens of people from all over the world, have many of them translated into Spanish, organize interviews, and put everything together in a uniform format. The minor typographical and translation errors that are seen in some parts of the book are understandable and forgivable in view of the magnitude of the task.

The book is organized into three sections: (1) articles by international experts in the field, intended to frame community interpreting in the context of Translation Studies; (2) contributions by experts in Spain, discussing specific settings where community interpreting is performed in that country; and (3) reports on community interpreting in 11 different countries and three regions of Spain, consisting of essays written by or interviews conducted with practitioners and researchers in each country or region.

The first article in Section 1 is by the editor of the volume, Carmen Valero Garcés. She discusses the different labels that have been given to this type of interpreting (a common topic in writings in this field because of the lack of agreement on terminology and scope, as in Mikkelson 1996 and Gentile 1997), and proposes the Spanish equivalent of the term "public service interpreting." She then presents a literature review, examines the history of this type of interpreting, and assesses the prevailing situation in various countries.

The next contribution is from Cynthia Miguélez, who focuses on the professionalization of community interpreting in the countries of the European Union. She also remarks on the controversy over what to call this activity, but decides to use the term most prevalent in the United States and Canada, "community interpreting," throughout her paper to set aside the debate until the issue is finally resolved elsewhere. Miguélez examines market difficulties, recognition of the profession, working conditions, and other issues of professionalization identified during a panel discussion at the conference in 2002. She concludes that court interpreters in Europe are slightly better off in this regard than other community interpreters, and they may be able to pave the way for future improvements.

Jan Cambridge then looks at healthcare interpreting in the United Kingdom, though most of the issues she raises apply to other countries as well. She discusses the use of volunteer interpreters, advocacy and impartiality, the modes of interpreting, the role of the healthcare interpreter, and challenges faced by interpreters. One innovative feature of this article is the graphic depiction of the different levels of vulgarity or profanity in the language that interpreters must deal with, a very useful teaching tool.

Ann Corsellis follows with an article on training service providers to work with interpreters. She presents information on how to assess their intercultural communication abilities and on encouraging institutions to hire bilingual providers. Fortunately for those who do not read Spanish, Corsellis has published extensively on this subject (Corsellis 1997, 2000).

The next article in this section is by Helge Niska and is very similar to the one contained in the 2002 conference proceedings. It deals with the principles of terminology, the work of terminologists, the compilation of terminology databases by interpreters, and the strategies used by interpreters when there is no equivalent in the target language for a term used by a speaker in the source language. He also discusses planning policy at the national level and standardization issues. Of particular interest are the appendices, which contain syllabi of terminology courses at different schools of interpreting.

The second section of the book, devoted to public service interpreting in Spain, begins with an article by Roberto Mayoral Asensio on trends in the court interpreting profession. He reports on changes in the languages and venues where court interpreters work due to new waves of immigration into Spain, and points out that academic institutions and professional associations have an obligation not only to their own graduates and members, but also to society to adapt to the changing needs of the profession in Spain. The next article analyzes the prevailing market for court interpreters. The author decries the widespread use of agencies at the expense of credentialed interpreters, and predicts a gloomy future for the profession unless judicial authorities accept their responsibility for ensuring that only qualified interpreters are hired for legal proceedings.

Manuel Feria García has written a fascinating article on the translation of personal documents for Moroccan immigrants and the problems that result when Spanish authorities request the wrong documents for the information they need to process immigration applications, due to their ignorance of Moroccan customs. Next is an article on the role of interpreters in criminal proceedings, which also presents ethical guidelines for interpreters and offers some illuminating statistics on the languages interpreted in Spain's courts. This is followed by a description of a program established to enable translating and interpreting students to gain practical experience by interpreting for the local police.

Carmen Valero Garcés then discusses the situation of hospital interpreting in her country, noting that Spain lags behind other nations that have longer traditions of serving as host countries for immigrants. She makes recommendations for the development of greater resources in this area. Two articles address the issue of interpreting for immigration proceedings, one outlining the pitfalls of interpreting in asylum hearings and the other describing the functions of the translation and interpreting service at an NGO that represents refugees and asylum seekers in Spain. The next article provides the perspective of the freelance interpreter working for agencies, and the section concludes with a piece on communication problems in a hospital in Madrid with a large immigrant patient load.

The third section of the book presents reports on community interpreting in specific countries and regions of Spain, many of them essays written by leading experts such as Uldis Ozolins, Franz Pöchhacker, and Erik Hertog. There are also interviews with individuals who are knowledgeable about the role and status of interpreters in their countries. As a whole, the reports provide a comprehensive overview of prevailing trends in this growing profession.

Taken as a whole, the conference proceedings and the follow-up book make a valuable contribution to our understanding of the community interpreting profession.

References

Corsellis, A. (1997). Training needs of public personnel working with interpreters. In S. E. Carr, R. Roberts, A. Dufour & D. Steyn (Eds.), *The critical link: Interpreters in the community*. Amsterdam/Philadelphia: John Benjamins, 77–89.

Corsellis, A. (2000). Turning good intentions into good practice. Enabling the public services to fulfill their responsibilities. In R. P. Roberts, S. E. Carr, D. Abraham & A. Dufour (Eds.), *The critical link 2: Interpreters in the community*. Amsterdam/Philadelphia: John Benjamins, 89–99.

Gentile, A. (1997). Community interpreting or not? Practices, standards and accreditation. In S. E. Carr, R. Roberts, A. Dufour & D. Steyn (Eds.), *The critical link: Interpreters in the community*. Amsterdam/Philadelphia: John Benjamins, 109–118.

Mikkelson, H. (1996). Community interpreting: An emerging profession. *Interpreting*. 1 (1), 125–129.

∼

Bernd Meyer. *Dolmetschen im medizinischen Aufklärungsgespräch. Eine diskursanalytische Untersuchung zur Wissensvermittlung im mehrsprachigen Krankenhaus.* Münster/New York/München/Berlin: Waxmann Verlag, 2004. 250 pp. ISBN 3-8309-1297-3. [Mehrsprachigkeit 13.]

Reviewed by Christina Schäffner

Community interpreting, or public service interpreting, has become the object of increasing interest in recent years, as evidenced, for example, in the Critical Link conferences and the subsequent publications (e.g. Roberts et al. 2000). Community interpreters normally work in environments where foreigners or individuals from minority groups interact with public authorities in a host country, and such environments have an impact on the interpreter's performance and status. In addition to dealing with linguistic aspects of the delivery, recent research has therefore focused on ethical and sociological issues.

The present book is a contribution to this growing body of research, with the focus on interpreting in medical settings. It is based on the author's doctoral dissertation, which was part of a larger project carried out within the Research Centre on Multilingualism (Sonderforschungsbereich 'Mehrsprachigkeit') at Hamburg University in Germany. The topic of Meyer's research is doctor-patient communication in hospitals mediated by ad hoc interpreters, i.e. bilingual nurses or relatives of the patient. The language pair examined is German and Portuguese. The data come from authentic interactions, more specifically, from briefings for informed consent ('diagnostisches Aufklärungsgespräch'), in which German doctors inform patients of Portuguese background about diagnostic procedures and the potential risks involved. The briefings were tape-recorded and transcribed, and German glosses are provided for the Portuguese extracts in the transcripts used for illustration in the book.

Meyer is interested in how knowledge is communicated in a bilingual context, in other words, in how well the interpreters succeed in transferring the doctor's expert discourse into the target language, Portuguese. There are eight chapters, followed by a list of tables and figures and the bibliography. An abstract in English is provided at the beginning of the book. The first chapter contextualises the research and gives a brief overview of aims, corpus, method and findings. The methodology applied to the data analysis is firmly grounded in functional-pragmatic discourse analysis as developed by Konrad Ehlich and Jochen Rehbein (the importance of these two discourse analysts for Meyer's work is also reflected in the fact that there are 18 entries for Ehlich and 20 for Rehbein in the bibliography).

After a brief overview in Chapter 2 of linguistic analyses of interpreting in hospitals done by other scholars and a presentation of key aspects of functional-pragmatic discourse analysis, Chapter 3 deals with the institutional setting and characteristic features of institutional communication in hospitals. Briefings for informed consent, which are part of a 'hyperpragmeme' diagnosis/therapy, form the empirical basis of the research. These briefings are presented as a specific type of discourse in the context of doctor-patient interaction. Their structure and purpose are determined by the institutional actions in which they are embedded, and thus, they are characterised by a particular, recurring pattern of communicative action.

Briefings for informed consent are then presented in their illocutionary and propositional dimensions in Chapter 4. In terms of the illocutionary structure, briefings are characterised by a combination of speech acts, of which 'announcing' the intended method and 'describing' how it will be performed are, among several other acts, considered to be constitutive for the achievement of institutional purposes. Announcing and describing are speech acts initiated by the doctor to orient the patient towards a professional plan. The patient's cooperation needs to be ensured and must be reflected in the speech act of 'agreeing' (i.e. consent) performed by the patient at the end of the interaction. In terms of the propositional structure, briefings for consent reflect the transfer of professional knowledge to the patient. Particular propositional elements play a specific role in this respect, as can be seen in the linguistic structures used to identify the speech acts themselves or their elements (e.g. mentioning the planned method, the medical instrument to be used, parts of the body, expected results). The doctor's talk is characterised as semi-professional talk, since by using both medical and everyday terms, doctors aim at ensuring the patient's cooperation by overcoming gaps in medical knowledge.

Of particular relevance in structuring the discourse are information sheets for patients ('Aufklärungsbogen'), which form the basis of propositional plans.

The following two chapters deal with the effects of interpreting on doctor-patient communication. The author presents findings of a comparative analysis of how the propositional plan of announcing (Chapter 5) and the propositional dimensions of describing the method (Chapter 6) are realised linguistically in the source texts and in the interpreted versions. The qualitative analysis reveals that ad hoc interpreters have difficulties in finding equivalent linguistic forms in the target language for some of the medical terms that are important for achieving communicative purposes in briefings for informed consent in diagnostic settings. Such difficulties are illustrated with reference to terms that designate the method as a whole (e.g. 'Magenspiegelung/gastroscopy', 'Lungenspiegelung/bronchoscopy'), parts of the body (e.g. 'Speiseröhre/esophagus') or instruments (e.g. 'Schlauch/tube') that are important for the communicative process. Meyer found that the untrained ad hoc interpreters use certain procedures to compensate for these difficulties, such as repeating the medical term in German ('insertional code-switching') or replacing it with non-terminological forms. Other actions by the interpreter are of an ancillary communicative nature, such as pointing at parts of the body as illustrated in the patient information sheet (e.g. 'Speiseröhre' — 'este canal aqui' and pointing to it on the page). In other cases, interpreters rendered unknown medical terms morpheme-by-morpheme into the target language, resulting in comprehension problems which disrupt the coherence of the doctor's discourse.

The results show that the processing of the source text information depends on the interpreter's own active participation in the triadic interaction in the institutional setting. That is, the interpreters' knowledge of the purpose and content of the briefing, their own knowledge of medical procedures, and their relationship to the main actors influence the strategies applied and the target-language words chosen. For example, insertional code-switching depends on the interaction between the ad hoc interpreter and the patient and requires the patient to have some knowledge of the source language. Interpreters also usually monitor the patient's understanding. In some cases, they ask patients if they have understood the message or a specific medical term. This happens often when the interpreter has translated a complex compound term morpheme-by-morpheme into the target language. Meyer also finds that even nurses who act as interpreters may find it difficult to designate parts of the body in their native Portuguese, if they had their professional training in Germany.

Chapter 7 then summarises the results and concludes that the quality of interpreted briefings for informed consent is left to chance and that, as a rule, the information provided to the patient is less accurate and complete if the interpreters are non-trained bilinguals. The very brief Chapter 8, 'Ausblick' (looking ahead), therefore argues for interpreter training that provides information about the communicative function of types of discourse, such as briefings for informed consent, and that such training should focus on those linguistic forms that play an important role in achieving the communicative purposes. There is, however, another important issue raised in this concluding chapter: Germany does not officially regard itself as a multilingual country, and consequently, migrants as well as doctors and nurses working in German hospitals are faced with problems caused by the linguistic barriers. In a political climate in which migrants are expected to learn the language of the host country, community interpreting done by qualified interpreters will not be high on the agenda. This is also the rather pessimistic conclusion with which Meyer ends the book.

Readers and scholars interested in ethical and sociological issues of interpreting in medical institutions will not find much information in the present book. As should have become clear, the research is more a contribution to functional-pragmatic discourse analysis (which is the author's disciplinary background) rather than to interpreting studies, which is also reflected in the fact that only less than 20 percent of the titles listed in the Bibliography belong to Translation and Interpreting Studies. There are a few issues of a sociological and ethical nature which are briefly hinted at and which would deserve more attention, for example, the face-saving strategies used by the ad hoc interpreters, the procedures for monitoring their own performance or their strategies for interacting with the patients (Meyer shows, for example, that relatives of the patients attempt to downplay or ignore possible negative aspects of the medical procedure in order to calm patients). The issue of the social status of interpreters in the eyes of the public authorities and the problems associated with using untrained interpreters in complex professional environments (see also Pöchhacker & Kadric 1999) cannot be dealt with on the basis of a detailed comparative discourse analysis alone.

There are many footnotes in this book, which is a characteristic feature of German doctoral dissertations. There are also a number of errors (the odd missing word and a relatively large number of typing errors), incorrect references to figures (Figure 2 is in Section 3.4.2 on p. 52 and not in Section 3.1.4 as stated on p. 49), missing information (on p. 220 there is a reference to an appendix which does not exist). These formal problems may be the result of the revision of the doctoral dissertation for book publication, but they should have been spotted in the editing process.

References

Pöchhacker, Franz & Kadric, Mira (1999). The hospital cleaner as healthcare interpreter. A case study. *The Translator* 5 (2), 161–178.
Roberts, Roda, Carr, Silvana E., Abraham, Diana & Dufour, Aideen (Eds.) (2000). *The Critical Link 2: Interpreters in the community.* Amsterdam/Philadelphia: Benjamins.

~

Claudia V. Angelelli. *Revisiting the interpreter's role. A study of conference, court, and medical interpreters in Canada, Mexico, and the United States.* Amsterdam/Philadelphia: John Benjamins, 2004. xv + 125 pp. ISBN 90-272-1671-1

Claudia V. Angelelli. *Medical interpreting and cross-cultural communication.* Cambridge: Cambridge University Press, 2004. xiii + 153 pp. ISBN 0-521-83026-5

Reviewed by Helen Slatyer

The role of the interpreter has been an important theme in research into the nature of community-based interpreting. The publication in the last two decades of the findings of a growing body of research which has analysed the discourse of interpreter-mediated interaction has led to increased acceptance of a more active role for interpreters in managing and coordinating talk. However, while a range of linguistic and interactional features of interpreter-mediated communication has been described, the interpersonal role of the interpreter as a social actor has attracted less systematic attention as the focus of research. It is this aspect of role which is the most complex and contentious, with an on-going debate about whether the interpreter should advocate for her clients and a lack of consensus in attributing the label of advocacy to behaviours in interpreting practice. There is a prevailing sense, though, that setting is a key component in defining this aspect of role, with the impression that prescriptive role models are more acceptable in legalistic settings and more latitude is appropriate for the medical setting.

In *Revisiting the interpreter's role* and *Medical interpreting and cross-cultural communication* Claudia Angelelli reports on two studies which use contrasting research methodologies (one quantitative, the other ethnographic) to provide two distinct perspectives on the role of the interpreter. Role definitions in the two studies are centred on the construct of visibility/invisibility in an attempt to dispel notions of interpreting — not only in community-based interpreting, but also in conference and court interpreting — which consider the interpreter as a non-participant (reflecting the much-maligned conduit metaphor). The research builds on existing work that explores interpreter-mediated communication from a range of linguistic and sociological perspectives to obtain a rich description of the interaction in its social and institutional context.

Angelelli's definition of visibility encompasses the linguistic elements of interpreted interactions as well as the interpersonal role of the interpreter, described according to five subcomponents: alignment with the parties; establishing trust with/facilitating mutual respect between the parties; communicating affect as well as message; explaining cultural gaps/interpreting culture as well as language; establishing communication rules during the conversation. These subcomponents of visibility reflect the points of tension between interpreters' prescribed roles based on the key principles of interpreters' codes of ethics (specifically the principles of impartiality and accuracy) and expectations and experience of roles in practice. Angelelli describes this tension as existing in a 'closed circle', where uninformed and untested models of practice are based on experiences of education (informed only by practice), professional practice, discourse about interpreting (within the profession) and the influence of professional associations. To break into this closed circle, she calls for models of practice that are informed by theory and research which draw on related disciplines such as linguistic anthropology, bilingualism, cross-cultural studies and social theory. It is these research-based theories and models of interpreting, along with the experience gained in practice, which should underpin the education of interpreters.

Revisiting the interpreter's role presents Angelelli's doctoral research: a survey study of conference, court and medical interpreters' views on their role. The main objective of the study was to investigate the extent to which interpreters perceived themselves as visible participants in the interpreter-mediated event and whether the setting in which they worked influenced their perception. The survey sought to determine: (1) whether a relationship exists between interpreters' social backgrounds and their perception of visibility; (2) where interpreters working in different settings fall on the continuum of visibility/invisibility for interpreter perceptions of role; and (3) whether interpreters working in different settings differ in their perceptions of role (p. 67).

In the first chapter, a brief outline of the historical development of the profession introduces the field. This historical overview encompasses evidence of dialogue interpreting in the ancient world and the use of interpreters by Columbus during the Spanish Conquest of the American continent through to the relatively more recent emergence of conference and court interpreting. The key issues discussed in this overview are the influence of the historical development of the profession on current practice, the predominant research paradigms in conference, court and community-based interpreting, the tension between prescribed and ac-tual roles and the range of metaphors used to describe role which tend to reinforce the notion of the interpreter as a non-participant. Angelelli considers why invis-ibility predominates as the model for practice and also touches briefly on issues re-lated to the training of interpreters and the influence of professional organisations in maintaining prescriptive models of role. The chapter concludes with a rationale for the study, elaborating on the "closed circle" described above. Angelelli argues for an interdisciplinary approach to the investigation of interpreting, allowing for a true understanding of the complexity of intercultural and interlinguistic com-munication which also takes into account the interpersonal forces at play within the interpreter-mediated encounter.

In Chapter 2 the theoretical underpinnings for this study are outlined. In order to understand the social role of the interpreter, Angelelli has sought relevant theo-ries from sociology (such as theory on impression formation, attribution theory, status of self/self-perception), social theory (Bourdieu's theory of practice) and linguistic anthropology. These theories contribute to a view of communication as a socially embedded activity within the institutional context in which it takes place and feed directly into the elaboration of the survey items. The development of the survey instrument, the Interpreter's Interpersonal Role Inventory (IPRI), is de-scribed in detail in Chapter 3. The development was meticulous, drawing on prin-ciples of survey design used in psychology to achieve a high degree of validity and reliability. Construct validation was conducted through reference to the literature in the field (research on the subcomponents of visibility outlined above) and by seeking expert opinions and holding focus groups. Eighty items were drafted and categorized according to Wadensjö's taxonomy of monologic and dialogic com-munication. They were equally distributed into beliefs about role (e.g. Item 57: "As an interpreter, I am the only party to the conversations who can control the flow of communication") and behaviour in practice (e.g. Item 61: "I actively work to keep the more dominant party from monopolizing the conversation"). The IPRI achieved a high degree of reliability (.90) and inter-item consistency on the pilot. The final version consisted of two parts: Part A containing 13 questions serving as background measures and targeting social factors (gender, age, socioeconomic status and education — general and related to interpreting); and Part B consisting of the 38 items to measure visibility. Responses to items were based on agreement/disagreement on a 6-point Likert scale (from "completely disagree" to "completely agree"). Some items tend to reflect the context of community-based interpreting more strongly (e.g. Item 29: "Sometimes interpreting tears is more necessary than interpreting the words that accompany them" or Item 34: "As an interpreter my role is to compensate for the power differential between the parties"). This was in fact picked up in the unsolicited comments from respondents (principally from the cohort of conference interpreters).

The administration and results of the survey are reported in Chapter 4. Once the validation process was complete, the IPRI was administered to the target population of conference, court and medical interpreters from Canada, the US and Mexico, who were recruited through professional organisations such as AIIC (Association Internationale des Interprètes de Conférence), NAJIT (National Association of Judiciary Interpreters and Translators) and organisations of healthcare interpreters or community interpreters. A random sample stratified by region and language was taken from the listings in the directories. 293 interpreters completed the survey, most of them (70%) females. The majority of respondents were 40–49 years old, with only 27% having formal education in interpreting. Most had followed at least some professional development and had between 5 and 10 years of experience in interpreting. Results indicate that interpreters see themselves as visible to a greater or lesser degree, with setting as the factor that is most strongly associated with self-perceptions of visibility for all five subcomponents. Not surprisingly, the medical interpreters saw themselves as the most visible, with court interpreters less so and conference interpreters as the least visible. Associations between socioeconomic background/or background measures were weakly supported, with no effect for level of education or gender, and with an effect for age, with the older interpreters seeing themselves as the least visible. Angelelli suggests that this may be evidence of the beginning of a shift in thinking due to the findings of research filtering through to practitioners.

By way of conclusion, Chapter 5 proposes a theory of interpreting as outlined in Chapter 2, confirming Angelelli's starting premise that an interdisciplinary approach is essential if we are to understand the complexity of the interpreter as a social entity. The implications of the findings of the study for education and professional organisations are also discussed with the possible applications of the IPRI. The final section reviews the construct of invisibility in light of the findings of the survey.

Three appendices are included: the final version of the IPRI (Appendix 1), the list of organisations contacted for distribution of the survey (Appendix 2) and a thoughtful letter from one respondent who is a conference interpreter and member of AIIC. The letter describes the writer's frustration at the lack of recognition, by educational institutions and the profession itself, of the role of the conference interpreter as an active and visible participant in the conference proceedings. This contrasts strongly with the content of the unsolicited comments.

This study is of interest for a number of reasons: firstly the careful design of the IPRI and the size of the cohort surveyed have yielded statistically significant findings to a question that had not previously been investigated in this manner. The fact that the findings support the hypotheses is not surprising, but the existence of solid empirical evidence for claims such as these provides a basis for argumentation for a change in how role is defined. Secondly, for the purposes of constructing the IPRI, invisibility has been unpacked in such a way as to make explicit the subcomponents of visibility reflecting both linguistic and social characteristics of the interpreter's participation. Lastly, the IPRI lends itself to administration in a range of contexts for a replication of the survey and can also be used as a background measure for qualitative research, as Angelelli herself has done in the second study reviewed here.

Medical interpreting and cross-cultural communication narrows and deepens the focus of enquiry into visibility to report on the findings of an ethnographic study into the interpreting service of a large hospital in California. This case study explores visibility through the discourse of interpreter-mediated communication in the hospital, triangulated with interview data, survey data and artefacts from the site, collected over a two-year period. The principal focus of enquiry is the role of the interpreter in interpreter-mediated communication in the context of the hospital interpreting service.

The rationale for the study overlaps somewhat with that of *Revisiting the interpreter's role*: the necessity of using an interdisciplinary approach in the investigation of interpreter roles, which accounts for the social involvement of the interpreter. In addition, one of the objectives of the study was to collect a large number of audio-recordings of interpreter-mediated events for the investigation.

The volume begins with a discussion of the literature on role, considering the tension between conduit models of interpreting (the interpreter as an invisible participant or non-participant) and actual roles observed in naturalistic data (interpreters as actively participating in the interaction) as one of the main dilemmas facing interpreters in their practice. The author reviews the growing body of discourse-based research on interpreter-mediated interaction in medical settings, citing authors who question dogmatic applications of codes of ethics in defining roles for medical interpreters. On this basis Angelelli proposes a model of "visible interpreters", whose role also includes: communicating cultural gaps and linguistic barriers; communicating affect and content; establishing trust; facilitating mutual respect; putting parties at ease during the conversation; creating more balance (or imbalance) during the conversation by aligning with one of the parties; advocating for or establishing alliances with either party; and managing the requested and given information. These functions are manifested in the data as: introducing or positioning the party to the interpreter-mediated event; setting communication rules (e.g. turn-taking) and controlling the traffic of information; paraphrasing or explaining terms or concepts; sliding messages up and down the register scale; filtering information; aligning with one of the parties; and replacing one of the parties (p. 11).

In Chapter 2 Angelelli discusses the nature of doctor-patient communication and the importance of establishing a positive, caring relationship with patients for positive health outcomes. Patient-centred approaches to medicine recognize the importance of dialogue as a means of building mutual understanding and collaboration between healthcare practitioners and their patients. Lexicogrammatical choices impact subtly on the success of the communication. Angelelli wonders how the interpreter fits into this model of care and what the consequences of the triadic relationship and the interpersonal role of the interpreter are, hence the importance of gaining a better understanding of the dynamics of interpreter-mediated healthcare communication.

The range of theoretical perspectives that have been taken to examine the role of the interpreter in this study are outlined in Chapter 3. Not surprisingly, there is considerable overlap with Chapter 2 of *Revisiting the interpreter's role,* as the theoretical framework established for the survey is also employed in this study, but implemented in a very different methodological framework (ethnography). Angelelli describes the theories from related disciplines as lenses through which the interpreter-mediated event is viewed. The use of a number of different lenses enables the researcher to identify aspects of the event which would normally be overlooked or misunderstood. In addition to social theory and sociology, linguistic anthropology, notably the work of Hymes, is also central to the understanding of communication in its social and cultural context. Angelelli elaborates on Hymes' taxonomy of notions of communication to contrast monolingual and interpreted communication in the hospital setting.

Chapter 4 describes the hospital in which the case study takes place, the role of the researcher and the details of the setting where the interpreters work. The hospital is described in relation to the town in which it is located and its demographics and history. The study set out to target Spanish-English interpreters, and the site chosen had the highest number of interpreters for this language pair (10 full-time and 3 part-time interpreters). The Interpreting Service offers both face-to-face and over-the-speakerphone interpreting, and both of these modes were included in the study. The ten interpreters that formed the focus of this study are described according to their age, level of education, seniority in the service, professional experience and ethnic background. None of them had been formally trained as interpreters, but they had been trained on the job by shadowing more experienced practitioners. The site where the service is located is described, as well as a typical day in the life of an interpreter in the service.

In Chapter 5 the data analysis is described. Consistent with ethnographic research, the report is descriptive, giving details about the collection of data and the findings from the analysis. The IPRI was completed by the interpreters and included in the study data. Artefacts such as notes sent between the interpreters and documentation originating from the service (health-related pamphlets, etc.) were collected. Audio-recordings of medical appointments, field notes and interviews were also part of this vast data set. The methods used for coding and analysis are described in detail, with samples of each type of data. Content analysis was conducted for the interviews. The naturalistic data of interpreter-mediated interactions was collected either directly from the speakerphone or through audio-recordings of the face-to-face interactions. The different types of events identified were categorized and the discourse analysed for evidence of visibility.

A total of 392 interpreter-mediated events was recorded. Of these, 378 are described as providing evidence of visibility, compared to only 14 where the interpreter seemed to be invisible. The majority (381) were conducted over the speakerphone. In Chapter 6 the data is discussed through a description of the categories and sub-categories of visibility that have been identified. Visibility is described as a continuum ranging from high visibility (complete text ownership, replacing the monolingual interlocutor) to low visibility (controlling the flow of traffic) and is aligned with the degree of consequence on the informational content of the encounter. Data samples are discussed to illuminate the criteria for categorizing events on the visibility continuum. Instances of minor visibility typically occur during the opening and closing phases of the interaction, where the interpreters introduce themselves or close the conversation with a formulaic expression such as "you're welcome". Instances of major visibility occur particularly in the discovery, examination and evaluation phases of the interaction. One of the samples cited has the interpreter cutting the patient's storytelling short to request that she simply reply to the doctor's question with a yes/no answer, and then lays down the ground rules for the control of the traffic. Another example of major visibility is during history-taking by a nurse. The nurse hands over responsibility for this to the interpreter, and the interpreter proceeds to ask the usual questions about chronic illness ("Have you ever been operated on or hospitalised?"). This results in an extended exchange between the interpreter and the patient over twenty turns with no intervention from the nurse until the interpreter concludes with a summary of the patient's responses. It appears from this sample that this is the nurse's expectation. Other evidence of major visibility is the conscious lowering of register to one that the interpreter perceives to be more appropriate for the patient.

The Interpreter Service manager and each of the interpreters was interviewed. The interview data is paraphrased and described in Chapter 7, with many examples from the data. The interviews encouraged interpreters to talk about their work, the people for whom they interpret, the challenges and stressful moments they must overcome and how they characterize their role. The interviews reflect a broad range of perceptions about role, from alignment with more prescriptive role models to justification for claiming authorship. Prominent in the interview data is awareness of the power differential between the healthcare providers and their patients and the position of the interpreter in reducing the gap. Many expressed the belief that they should change register to make the patient feel more comfortable. Another frequent comment was that the doctors did not have much time, and in order for the patient to get the most out of the meeting, the interpreters needed to control the flow of traffic and filter the information or paraphrase. The Interpreter Service manager strongly believed that these strategies were necessary to meet the communicative goals of the encounter.

Chapter 8 concludes the volume with a discussion of the role metaphors that the interpreters use to describe their role and the functions they carry out in the context of that role. These role metaphors describe the interpreter's agency in achieving the communicative goals of the encounter by seeking information or evaluating the worth of what is said. A final section discusses the theoretical and practical implications of the findings and the importance of considering the interpreter as a social actor.

These two volumes by Angelelli make a valuable contribution to our understanding of roles in interpreter-mediated interaction. Visibility is a complex construct which incorporates a range of linguistic and interpersonal features encompassing the ethical principles of accuracy (in managing and coordinating talk) and impartiality (in aligning with one or another of the parties). The two studies are complementary in providing contrasting perspectives on how interpreters view their participation in interpreter-mediated interaction. The importance of gaining greater awareness of the social aspect of role is demonstrated by the data samples and by the voices of the interpreters in their interviews and comments, as they discuss their role and justify the strategies that they employ in their interpreting. This is how they contribute to achieving the communicative goals of the healthcare providers and their patients.

In the series *Benjamins Current Topics (BCT)* the following titles have been published thus far or are scheduled for publication: